OUR MISSION

The mission of *Bridging The Gap Foundation* is to improve reproductive health and contraceptive decision making of women and men by providing up-to-date educational resources to the physicians, nurses and public health leaders of tomorrow.

OUR VISION

Our vision is to provide educational resources to the health care providers of tomorrow to help ensure informed choices, better service, access, happier and more successful contraceptors, competent clinicians, fewer unintended pregnancies and disease prevention.

Examples of questions answered on this website:

- If a woman's severe migraine headaches stop completely on combined pills, can she continue taking pills even though the World Health Organization recommends that combined pills not be used with her type of headaches?
- Do birth control pills cause breast cancer? (Marchbanks 2002 update) ◄

To medical students, residents and nurse practitioners receiving this book...please send us your comments by visiting our web site.

.com

D0974114

IMPORTANT DISCLAIMER

The authors remind readers that this book is intended to educate health care providers, not guide individual therapy. The authors advise a person with a particular problem to consult a primary-care clinician or a specialist in obstetrics, gynecology, or urology (depending on the problem or the contraceptive) as well as the product package insert and other references before diagnosing, managing, or treating the problem. Under no circumstances should the reader use this handbook in lieu of or to override the judgment of the treating clinician. The order in which diagnostic or therapeutic measures appear in this text is not necessarily the order that clinicians *should* follow in each case. The authors and staff are not liable for errors or omissions.

Sixth Edition, 2003-2004
ISBN 0-9638875-2-1
Printed in the United States of America
The Bridging the Gap Foundation

On 216 pages, we cannot possibly provide you with all the information you might want or need about contraception. Many of the questions clinicians ask are answered in the textbook *Contraceptive Technology* or in detail on our website. Visit us regularly at:

www.managingcontraception.com

A POCKET GUIDE TO

MANAGING CONTRACEPTION

2003-2004 Edition

Robert A. Hatcher, MD, MPH
Professor of Gynecology and Obstetrics
Emory University School of Medicine

Anita L. Nelson, MD
Professor of Obstetrics and Gynecology
David Geffen School of Medicine at UCLA
Harbor-UCLA Medical Center

Miriam Zieman, MD
Associate Professor of Gynecology and Obstetrics
Emory University School of Medicine

Philip D. Darney, MD, MSc
Professor of Obstetrics, Gynecology and Reproductive Sciences
University of California, San Francisco
San Francisco General Hospital

Mitchell D. Creinin, MD
Associate Professor of Obstetrics, Gynecology and Reproductive Sciences
University of Pittsburgh School of Medicine
Magee-Womens Hospital

Harriet R. Stosur, MD
Clinician in Obstetrics and Gynecology, Northwest Permanente
Portland, Oregon

Carrie Cwiak, MD
Assistant Professor of Gynecology and Obstetrics
Emory University School of Medicine

Technical and Computer Support:
Anna Poyner, Daniel Skelton, Max Harrell, Don Bagwell
Digital Impact Design, Inc., Cornelia, Georgia

Special Thanks: Copies of *A Pocket Guide to Managing Contraception* are being sent to all medical students in the United States and to residents and faculty in Family Medicine and in Obstetrics and Gynecology. They are available thanks to the David and Lucile Packard Foundation. Thanks to Duramed, Berlex, Organon, Parke Davis and Wyeth, it has also been possible to provide 200,000 copies of this book to nurses, nurse practitioners and nursing students. We are extremely grateful. If you know of a class of medical students or a group of residents who have not received copies of this book, please notify us at our website www.managingcontraception.com or call 706-265-7435.

The Bridging the Gap Foundation • Tiger, Georgia

Dear Colleagues and Friends:

➤ As the cover suggests, the new options continue! Last year it was **Mirena**, the levonorgestrel intrauterine contraceptive, **Lunelle**, the **NuvaRing**, **Yasmin** and the **Ortho Evra Patch.** This year it is a new sterilization technique that may be important in the delivery of sterilization services for women, **Essure**; **Seasonale**, the combined pill a woman takes for ◄ 84 days before a hormone-free interval; and **advanced prescription of Plan B**. There is ◄ more on **Mirena** use in the treatment of menorrhagia and DUB. ◄

This is the sixth edition of *A Pocket Guide to Managing Contraception*. Thanks to the generosity of the David and Lucile Packard Foundation, all U.S. medical students and residents in Obstetrics and Gynecology and Family Medicine programs throughout the country have been provided the last four editions of this pocket guide. Over 200,000 nurses and nursing students and thousands of advanced care providers have also received copies of *Managing Contraception*. As of mid-June 2003, very close to 634,000 copies of the six ◄ editions of *Managing Contraception* will be in circulation.

Managing Contraception was developed as a way to put practical information about birth control and STIs into students' and residents' hands and pockets at the time they need contraception personally as well as information about contraception for patients! *Contraceptive Technology*, a much longer text, has matured over the course of its 18 editions into a comprehensive reference book that provides essential, readable information about contraceptive management, reproductive health issues, population dynamics, STIs and sexuality issues. To complement *Contraceptive Technology*, we have created this lightweight, pocket-sized handbook to meet the immediate needs of medical and nursing students, residents, physicians and other health care providers. Our target audiences praise the clarity of flow charts, the practical suggestions, color photos of the various pills, the CDC STI Treatment Guidelines (now updated to the 2002 guidelines), and the small size! For the convenience of our readers, information that has been added since the last edition of *Managing Contraception* is easy to find. Just look for an arrow! ➤ or ◄

Robert A. Hatcher

Robert A. Hatcher, MD, MPH
Professor of Gynecology and Obstetrics
Emory University School of Medicine
Atlanta, Georgia
President, The Bridging the Gap Foundation

We dedicate this edition of **Managing Contraception** to
John D. Thompson, MD ←

"Voluntary family planning is important for the health of women, children and families," John D. Thompson repeated this phrase often, arguing that no other explanation need be tendered to justify a commitment of time and financial resources to the delivery of completely voluntary birth control services. Forget the argument that smaller families could be good for the economics of a family. Forget the argument that women deserve the right to choose to control their own reproductive destinies. Forget the arguments that there is a world population problem or that population control could be good for the environment. *"Family planning is important simply because voluntary family planning is important for the health of women, children and families,"* he would say.

Dan Thompson was a superb surgeon and the care he lavished on individual women was legion. This was known by every faculty member, resident and medical student in the Department of Gynecology and Obstetrics at the Emory University School of Medicine in Atlanta. He chaired this department for 25 years. It was also known by specialists in gynecology and obstetrics across the land. As the senior author of the widely used text, *TeLinde's Operative Gynecology*, John D. Thompson's pursuit of excellence and efforts to share the most up-to-date information with professional colleagues had an international impact. But **JDT** had another side less typical of medical school leaders.

In an era when research, research, research was the focus of attention ("publish or perish") for most medical school professors, and public health was so low on the list of priorities for the chairmen (most were men) of most medical school departments, Dan Thompson focused on Pap smears for the prevention of cervical cancer for *all women in Georgia*, voluntary family planning *for all women in Georgia*; and quality antepartum services for *high risk women throughout the state of Georgia.*

Inspired by Dr. Mary Calderone, Medical Director of the Planned Parenthood Federation of America and Alexander D. Langmuir, head of the Epidemic Intelligence Service at the CDC, Dan Thompson set out to make voluntary contraceptive services available to all women who wanted them in Atlanta. The first full-time physician sponsored by the federal government was Dr. Nicholas Wright. He was assigned to work with Dr. Thompson at Grady. The next EIS officer assigned to family planning was Dr. Carl W. Tyler, also assigned to work with Dr. Thompson at Grady. Carl went on to develop the CDC's remarkable Division of Reproductive Health. Much of the early contraceptive research and many quality service programs can be attributed to the work of CDC physicians and nurses trained under Carl Tyler, Roger Rochat and Carol Hogue.

Thank you, Dan Thompson, for the immense contributions you have made on behalf of women seeking voluntary contraceptive, sterilization and abortion services.

ii

Many have contributed their sensitivity, time, graphics and layout skills, financial support, friendship, encouragement, patience and love in the creation of this ***Pocket Guide to Managing Contraception***. This book has been a labor of love. We have tried to condense our thoughts into a format that clinicians and counselors can carry in their pockets. Gems have come to us from many corners of the world. We thank all contributors, including:

- **Jeffrey Allen,** superb, caring breast radiologist at Piedmont Hospital in Atlanta and contributing artist to *MC*
- **Felix Andarsio,** a fine former chief resident in obstetrics and gynecology at Emory University
- **Marcia Ann Angle,** committed international leader in the quest for high quality reproductive health services at Intrah at University of North Carolina (UNC), Chapel Hill
- **Kaea Beresford,** Gyn-Ob resident at Emory University
- **Rachel Blankstein,** author of pilot edition of *MC* and Peace Corps volunteer in Niger; Johns Hopkins nursing school student
- **Stephen F. Brandt,** resident in internal medicine; has deep reservoirs of concern and caring; and great attention to detail
- **Sharon L. Camp,** president, Women's Capital Corporation, the company that produces and distributes PLAN B
- **Martha Campbell** and the David and Lucile Packard Foundation, made *MC* possible
- **Willard Cates,** president, Family Health International, researcher in contraception, STIs and HIV, and author of *Contraceptive Technology*; cheerleader!
- **Preeti Loomba Chada,** Technical Assistant Director, Clinical Affairs Division at Ortho-McNeil
- **Camaryn Chrisman,** medical student at Wake Forest, author of articles on WHO Medical Eligibility Criteria
- **Sarah Clark** and staff in the Population Program at the David and Lucile Packard Foundation. Their support of this book from the very start made this effort a reality
- **Kathryn M. Curtis,** Women's Health and Fertility Branch, CDC; author of articles on WHO Medical Eligibility Criteria
- **Anne Lange-Dunlop,** researcher on fertility awareness methods. Family practice faculty, Emory University School of Medicine
- **Alison Edelman,** family planning fellow, Department of Obstetrics and Gynecology, Oregon Health and Sciences University
- **Susan Eisendrath,** reproductive health initiative director at the American Medical Women's Association; has developed a marvelous reproductive health curriculum for medical schools
- **Michelle Fox,** family planning fellow at the University of Pittsburgh School of Medicine
- **Erica Frank,** preventionist, environmentalist and associate professor of family and preventive medicine and anatomy at Emory University
- **Diana Frost,** Manager, Medical Education at Ortho-McNeil and enthusiastic supporter of nurse practitioners
- **Timothy Grimes,** Director of Professional Education and Scientific Affairs at Ortho-McNeil
- **Felicia Guest,** AIDS educator, wise observer and an author of *Contraceptive Technology*
- **John Guillebaud,** professor of family planning and reproductive health at University College London Hospitals and medical director of the Margaret Pyke Center for Study and

Training in Family Planning. We thank John for permission to use information from *Contraception Today* (Martin Dunitz Ltd.), London, in *MC*

- **Melissa Halbach**, Gyn-Ob resident at Emory University
- **Peter Hatcher**, family practice physician, Multnomah County HD, Portland, Oregon; lover of gardening, photography, his family and dogs and a loyal friend
- **Wanjiku Kabiru**, maternal and fetal medicine fellow at Emory University
- **Andrew Kaunitz**, professor and assistant chair, OB/GYN department, University of Florida; Health Sciences Center, Jacksonville, Florida
- **Maxine Keel,** administrative assistant at the Emory University Family Planning Program, dreamer, inspiration and friend
- **Bert Peterson,** contraceptive research leader at the CDC in Atlanta and at the WHO in Geneva; former gynecology professor at Emory (see dedication in 2001-2002)
- **Erika Pluhar,** author of *A Personal Guide to Managing Contraception, SE101* Dissertation in human sexuality on mother/daughter communication
- **Malcolm Potts**, perhaps the most creative force in the field of family planning, human sexuality and reproductive health. Students at U.C. Berkeley love him
- **Anna Poyner**, graphic artist who designed every page in this book; Digital Impact Design in Cornelia, Georgia
- **Dian "Tossy" Hitt Sanders,** resident in gynecology and obstetrics at Emory University ◄—
- **Sharon Schnare,** dreamer, nurse practitioner and nurse midwife consultant and trainer in Seattle; remarkable teacher
- **Felicia Stewart,** Adjunct Professor of Obstetrics and Gynecology at the University of California in San Francisco; strong believer that both the disadvantages and advantages of each method need to be aired. So much help on the NuvaRing chapter
- **Stephanie B. Teal,** family planning fellow and clinical instructor in department of ◄— obstetrics and gynecology; New York Presbyterian Hospital
- **Ian Tilley,** positive, constructive resident in gynecology and obstetrics at Emory University ◄—
- **Andrea Tone,** historian in the Department of History, Technology and Society at Georgia Tech, Atlanta; specializing in the history of contraception
- **James Trussell,** an author of *Contraceptive Technology* who developed the failure rates and cost figures used throughout *MC*; champion of emergency contraception
- **Marcel Vekemans,** a family planning specialist from Belgium working at INTRAH whose attention to detail improved this book so much
- **Jane Wamsher,** nurse practitioner at Grady Memorial Hospital in Atlanta; provided practical protocols and creative techniques for using book to teach
- **Lee Warner**, CDC researcher working on STDs and HIV; so much help on the condom chapters
- **Elisa S. Wells,** senior program officer at PATH; emergency contraception expert
- **Aisha Woodard,** Gyn-Ob resident at Emory University
- **Honor Woodard,** contraceptive information specialist at Bridging the Gap Foundation; editor of *MC*
- **Kim Workowski,** CDC researcher on STDs and HIV; so much help on 2002 update of CDC STD Guidelines
- **Susan Wysocki,** strong public advocate for excellent women's health services
- **Edio J. Zampaglione,** associate director of contraception; Organon Pharmaceuticals, Inc. ◄—

ABBREVIATIONS USED IN THIS BOOK

ACOG	American College of Obstetricians & Gynecologists	**EE**	Ethinyl estradiol
		EPA	Environmental Protection Agency
AIDS	Acquired immunodeficiency syndrome	**ERT**	Estrogen replacement therapy
		ET	Estropey therapy
AMA	American Medical Association	**FAM**	Fertility awareness methods
ASAP	As soon as possible	**FDA**	Food and Drug Administration
BBT	Basal body temperature	**FH**	Family History
BCA	Bichloroacetic acid	**FSH**	Follicle stimulating hormone
BP	Blood pressure	**GAPS**	Guidelines for Adolescent Preventive Services
BTB	Breakthrough bleeding		
BTL	Bilateral tubal ligation	**GC**	Gonococcus/gonorrhea
BV	Bacterial vaginosis	**GI**	Gastrointestinal
CA	Cancer	**GnRH**	Gonadotrophin-releasing hormone
CDC	Centers for Disease Control and Prevention		
		HBsAg	Hepatitis B surface antigen
COCs	Combined oral contraceptives (estrogen & progestin)	**HBV**	Hepatitis B virus
		HCG	Human chorionic gonadotrophin
CMV	Cytomegalovirus		
CT	Chlamydia trachomatis	**HCV**	Hepatitis C virus
D & C	Dilation and curettage	**HDL**	High density lipoprotein
DCBE	Double contrast barium enema	**HIV**	Human immunodeficiency virus
DMPA	Depot-medroxyprogesterone acetate (Depo-Provera)	**HPV**	Human papillomavirus
		HRT	Hormone replacement therapy (estrogen & progestin)
DUB	Dysfunctional uterine bleeding		
DVT	Deep vein thrombosis	**HSV**	Herpes simplex virus (I or II)
E	Estrogen	**HT**	Hormone therapy
EC	Emergency contraception	**IM**	Intramuscular
ECPs	Emergency contraceptive pills ("morning-after pills")	**IPPF**	International Planned Parenthood Federation
ED	Erectile dysfunction	**IUC**	Intrauterine contraceptive
E₂	Estradiol	**IUD**	Intrauterine device
		IUP	Intrauterine pregnancy

v

IUS	Intrauterine system		PLISSIT	Permission giving
IV	Intravenous			Limited information
KOH	Potassium hydroxide			Simple suggestions
LAM	Lactational amenorrhea method			Intensive
LDL	Low-density lipoprotein			Therapy
LGV	Lymphogranuloma venereum		PMDD	Premenstrual dysphoric disorder
LH	Luteinizing hormone		PMS	Premenstrual syndrome
LMP	Last menstrual period		po	Latin: "per os"; orally
LNg	Levonorgestrel ←		POCs	Progestin-only contraceptives
MI	Myocardial infarction		POP	Progestin-only pill (minipill)
MIS	Misoprostol		PP	Postpartum
MMPI	Minnesota Multiphasic Personality Inventory		PPFA	Planned Parenthood Federation of America
MMWR	Mortality and Morbidity Weekly Report		PRN	As needed ←
			RR	Relative risk
MPA	Medroxyprogesterone acetate		Rx	Treatment
MTX	Methotrexate		SAB	Spontaneous abortion
MVA	Manual vacuum aspiration		SHBG	Sex hormone binding globulin
N-9	Nonoxynol-9 ←		SSRI	Selective Serotonin Reuptake Inhibitors ←
NFP	Natural family planning			
NSAID	Nonsteroidal anti-inflammatory drug		STD	Sexually transmitted disease
			STI	Sexually transmitted infection
OA	Overeaters Anonymous		Sx	Symptoms
OB/GYN	Obstetrics & Gynecology		TAB	Therapeutic abortion / ← elective abortion
OC	Oral contraceptive			
OR	Operating Room		TB	Tuberculosis
P	Progesterone		TCA	Trichloroacetic acid
Pap	Papanicolaou		TSS	Toxic shock syndrome
PCOS	Polycystic ovarian syndrome		URI	Upper respiratory infection
PE	Pulmonary embolism		UTI	Urinary tract infection
PET	Polyesther (fibers)		VTE	Venous thromboembolism
PG	Prostaglandin ←		VVC	Vulvovaginal candidiasis
pH	Hydrogen ion concentration		WHO	World Health Organization
PID	Pelvic inflammatory disease		ZDV	Zidovudine

1. Carry it with you. Arrows are a simple way for you to find the new information in this edition: ➡ or ⬅

2. Chapter 35 is taken directly from the most recent CDC recommended guidelines for the treatment of STIs.

3. Color photos of pills will help you to determine the pill your patient is/was on (A18 - A24)

4. The pages on the menstrual cycle concisely explain a very complicated series of events. Study pages 1-4 over and over again. Favorite subjects for exams!

5. Algorithms throughout book; several that might help you are on the following pages:
   • Page 106: Choosing a pill
   • Page 107: What to do about breakthrough bleeding or spotting on pills
   • Page 128: What to do if a woman returns late for her Depo-Provera injection

➡ 6. If you know the page number for the 2002-2003 edition, the information in your 2003-2004 book is likely to be on *approximately* the same page.

7. Use the listing of subjects on the back cover. It is the fastest way to get to the pages you want.

IMPORTANT PHONE NUMBERS

TOPIC	ORGANIZATION	PHONE NUMBER
Abortion	Abortion Hotline (NAF)	800-772-9100
Abuse/Rape	National Committee to Prevent Child Abuse	(312) 663-3520
	Coalition on Domestic Violence	800-537-2238
	CDC Rape Hotline (RAIN)	800-656-4673
		800-344-7432 Spanish
		800-243-7889
Adoption	Adopt a Special Kid-America	(202) 857-9708
	Adoptive Families of America	(651) 644-5223
Breastfeeding	La Leche League	800-LA-LECHE
Contraception	Planned Parenthood	800-230-7526
	Family Health International	(919) 544-7040
	PPFA	(212) 541-7800
Counseling	Peer Counseling for Gay/Lesbian	800-969-6884
	Peer Listening Line Gay/Lesbian	800-399-7337
	Depression after Delivery	800-944-4773
Emergency	Emergency Contraception Information	888-NOT-2-LATE
contraception	Plan B	800-330-1271
	Preven	888-PREVEN2
HIV/AIDS	CDC AIDS Hotline	800-342-2437
	CDC National AIDS Clearinghouse	800-458-5231
	AIDS Clinical Trials Information Service	800-874-2572
Pregnancy	Lamaze International	800-368-4404
STIs	Hepatitis B Coalition	(651) 647-9009
	CDC Sexually Transmitted Disease	800-227-8922
	Herpes and HPV Hotline	800-230-6039
	HELPline (Possible Workplace Exposure to HIV)	888-HIV-4911
		888-448-4911

Recommended Screening/Risk Assessment by Age**

AGES 13-18 YEARS

SCREENING

History
- Reason for visit
- Health status: medical, surgical, family
- Dietary/nutrition assessment
- Physical activity
- Use of complementary and alternative medicine
- Tobacco, alcohol, other drug use
- Abuse/neglect
- Sexual practices

Physical Examination
- Height
- Weight
- Blood pressure
- Secondary sexual characteristics (Tanner staging)
- Pelvic examination (yearly when sexually active or by age 18)
- Skin*

LABORATORY TESTS

Periodic
- Pap test (if sexually active or by age 18)

High-Risk Groups ★
- Hemoglobin level assessment
- Bacteriuria testing
- STI testing
- HIV testing
- Genetic testing/counseling
- Rubella titer assessment
- Tuberculosis skin test
- Lipid profile assessment
- Fasting glucose
- Cholesterol testing
- Hepatitis C virus testing
- Colorectal cancer screening

EVALUATION AND COUNSELING

Sexuality
- Development
- High-risk behaviors
- Preventing unwanted/unintended pregnancy
  Postponing sexual involvement
  Contraceptive options
- STIs
  Partner selection
  Barrier protection

Fitness and Nutrition
- Dietary/nutritional assessment (including eating disorders)
- Exercise: discussion of program
- Folic acid supplementation (0.4 mg/d)
- Calcium intake

Psychosocial Evaluation
- Interpersonal/family relationships
- Sexual identity
- Personal goal development
- Behavioral/learning disorders
- Abuse/neglect
- Satisfactory school experience
- Peer relationships

Cardiovascular Risk Factors
- Family history
- Hypertension
- Dyslipidemia
- Obesity
- Diabetes mellitus

Health/Risk Behaviors
- *Hygiene (including dental); fluoride supplementation*
- Injury prevention
  - Safety belts and helmets
  - Recreational hazards
  - Firearms
  - Hearing
- Skin exposure to ultraviolet rays
- Suicide: depressive symptoms
- Tobacco, alcohol, other drug use

IMMUNIZATIONS

Periodic
- Tetanus-diphtheria booster (once between ages 11 and 16 years)
- Hepatitis B vaccine (one series for those not previously immunized)

High-Risk Groups ★
- Influenza vaccine
- Hepatitis A vaccine
- Pneumococcal vaccine
- Measles, mumps, rubella vaccine
- Varicella vaccine

Leading Causes of Death:
- Motor vehicle accidents
- Homicide
- Suicide
- Cancer
- All other accidents and adverse effects
- Diseases of the heart
- Congenital anomalies
- Chronic obstructive pulmonary diseases

**Many organizations have screening guidelines. These are reprinted with permission from the American College of Obstetricians and Gynecologists from *Precis, Primary and Preventive Care: An Update in Obstetrics and Gynecology.* 1998. Revised December, 2000; ACOG Committee Opinion No 246.

5

Leading Causes of Morbidity:
- Acne
- Asthma
- Chlamydia
- Depression
- Dermatitis
- Headaches
- Infective, viral, and parasitic diseases
- Influenza
- Injuries
- Nose, throat, ear and upper respiratory infections
- Sexual assault
- Sexually transmitted deseases
- Urinary tract infections

Please see page 10 for High-Risk Factors

AGES 19-39 YEARS

SCREENING
History
- Reason for visit
- Health status: medical, surgical, family
- Dietary/nutrition assessment
- Physical activity
- Use of complementary and alternative medicine
- Tobacco, alcohol, other drug use
- Abuse/neglect
- Sexual practices
- Urinary and fecal incontinence

Physical Examination
- Height
- Weight
- Blood pressure
- Neck, adenopathy, thyroid
- Breasts
- Abdomen
- Pelvic examination
- Skin*

LABORATORY TESTING
Periodic
- Pap test (physician and patient discretion after three consecutive normal tests if low risk)

For High-Risk Groups *
- Hemoglobin level assessment
- Bacteriuria testing
- Mammography
- Fasting glucose test
- Cholesterol testing
- STI testing
- HIV testing
- Genetic testing/counseling
- Rubella titer assessment
- Tuberculosis skin testing
- Lipid profile assessment
- Thyroid-stimulating hormone testing
- Hepatitis C virus testing
- Colorectal cancer screening

EVALUATION AND COUNSELING
Sexuality
- High-risk behaviors
- Contraceptive options for prevention of unwanted pregnancy
- Preconceptional and genetic counseling for desired pregnancy
- STIs
  - Partner selection
  - Barrier protection
- Sexual function

Fitness and Nutrition
- Dietary/nutritional assessment
- Exercise: discussion of program
- Folic acid supplementation (0.4 mg/d)
- Calcium intake

Psychosocial Evaluation
- Interpersonal/family relationships
- Domestic violence
- Work satisfaction
- Lifestyle/stress
- Sleep disorders

Cardiovascular Risk Factors
- Family history
- Hypertension
- Dyslipidosis
- Obesity
- Diabetes mellitus
- Lifestyle

Health/Risk Behaviors
- Hygiene (including dental)
- Injury prevention
  - Safety belts and helmets
  - Occupational hazards
  - Recreational hazards
  - Firearms
  - Hearing
- Breast self-examination
- Chemoprophylaxis for breast cancer (for high-risk women ages 35 years or older)
- Skin exposure to ultraviolet rays
- Suicide: depressive symptoms
- Tobacco, alcohol, other drug use

IMMUNIZATIONS
Periodic
- Tetanus-diphtheria booster (every 10 years)

For High-Risk Factors *
- Measles, mumps, rubella vaccine
- Hepatitis A vaccine
- Hepatitis B vaccine
- Influenza vaccine
- Pneumococcal vaccine
- Varicella vaccine

Please see page 10 for High-Risk Factors

Leading Causes of Death:
- Accidents and adverse effects
- Cancer
- HIV infection
- Diseases of the heart
- Homicide
- Suicide
- Cerebrovascular disease
- Chronic liver disease and cirrhosis

Leading Causes of Morbidity:
- Asthma
- Back symptoms
- Breast disease
- Deformity or orthopedic impairment
- Depression
- Diabetes
- Gynecologic disorders
- Headache/migraines
- Hypertension
- Infective, viral, and parasitic diseases
- Influenza
- Injuries
- Nose, throat, ear, and upper respiratory infections
- Sexual assault/domestic violence
- Sexually transmitted diseases
- Skin rash/dermatitis
- Substance abuse
- Urinary tract infections
- Vaginitis

AGES 40-64 YEARS

SCREENING

History
- Reason for visit
- Health status: medical, surgical, family
- Dietary/nutrition assessment
- Physical activity
- Use of complementary and alternative medicine
- Tobacco, alcohol, and other drug use
- Abuse/neglect
- Sexual practices
- Urinary and fecal incontinence

Physical Examination
- Height, Weight, Blood pressure
- Oral cavity, Neck: adenopathy, thyroid
- Breasts, Axillae, Abdomen, Pelvic examination
- Skin*

LABORATORY TESTING

Periodic
- Pap test (physician and patient discretion after three consecutive normal tests if low risk)
- Mammography (every 1-2 years until age 50, yearly beginning at age 50)
- Cholesterol (every 5 yrs beginning at age 45)

- Yearly fecal occult blood testing plus flexible sigmoidoscopy every 5 years or colonoscopy every 10 years or double contrast barium enema (DCBE) every 5-10 years, with digital rectal examination performed at the time of each screening sigmoidoscopy, colonoscopy, or DCBE (beginning at age 50)
- Fasting glucose testing (every 3 years after age 45)

High-Risk Groups *
- Hemoglobin level assessment
- Bacteriuria testing
- Fasting glucose testing
- STI testing
- HIV testing
- Tuberculosis skin testing
- Lipid profile assessment
- Thyroid-stimulating hormone testing
- Hepatitis C virus testing
- Colorectal cancer screening

EVALUATION AND COUNSELING

Sexuality+
- High-risk behaviors
- Contraceptive options for prevention of unwanted pregnancy
- STIs
    Partner selection
    Barrier protection
- Sexual function

Fitness and Nutrition
- Dietary/nutrition assessment
- Exercise: discussion of program
- Folic acid supplementation (0.4 mg/d before age 50 years), Calcium intake

Psychosocial Evaluation
- Family relationships, Domestic violence
- Work satisfaction, Retirement planning
- Lifestyle/stress, Sleep disorders

Cardiovascular Risk Factors
- Family history
- Hypertension
- Dyslipidemia
- Obesity
- Diabetes mellitus
- Lifestyle

Health/Risk Behaviors
- Hygiene (including dental)
- Hormone replacement therapy
- Injury prevention
    - Safety belts and helmets
    - Occupational hazards
    - Recreational hazards
    - Sports involvement
    - Firearms
    - Hearing

+Preconceptional counseling is appropriate for certain women in this age group.

* Please see page 10 for High Risk Factors.

- Breast self-examination
- Chemoprophylaxis for breast cancer (for high risk women)
- Skin exposure to ultraviolet rays
- Suicide: depressive symptoms
- Tobacco, alcohol, other drug use

IMMUNIZATIONS
Periodic
- Influenza vaccine (annually beginning at age 50)
- Tetanus-diphtheria booster (every 10 yrs)
High-Risk Groups *
- Measles, mumps, rubella vaccine
- Hepatitis A vaccine, Hepatitis B vaccine
- Influenza vaccine, Pneumococcal vaccine
- Varicella vaccine

Leading Causes of Death:
- Cancer
- Diseases of the heart
- Cerebrovascular diseases
- Accidents and adverse effects
- Chronic obstructive pulmonary disease
- Diabetes mellitus
- Chronic liver disease and cirrhosis
- Pneumonia and influenza

Leading Causes of Morbidity:
- Arthritis/osteoarthritis
- Asthma
- Back symptoms
- Breast disease
- Cardiovascular disease
- Carpal tunnel syndrome
- Deformity or orthopedic impairment
- Depression
- Diabetes
- Headache
- Hypertension
- Infective, viral, and parasitic diseases
- Influenza
- Injuries
- Menopause
- Nose, throat, and upper respiratory infections
- Obesity
- Skin conditions/dermatitis
- Substance abuse
- Urinary tract infections
- Urinary tract (other conditions including urinary incontinence)
- Vision impairment

AGE 65 YEARS AND OLDER
SCREENING
History
- Reason for visit
- Health status: medical, surgical, family
- Dietary/nutritional assessment
- Physical activity
- Use of complementary and alternative medicine
- Tobacco, alcohol, other drug use, and concurrent medication use
- Abuse/neglect
- Sexual practices
- Urinary and fecal incontinence
Physical Examination
- Height, Weight, Blood pressure
- Oral cavity,
- Neck: adenopathy, thyroid
- Breasts, axillae
- Abdomen
- Pelvic examination
- Skin*

LABORATORY TESTING
Periodic
- Pap testing (physician and patient discretion after three consecutive normal tests if low risk)
- Urinalysis
- Mammography
- Cholesterol testing (every 3-5 years before age 75 years)
- Yearly fecal occult blood testing plus flexible sigmoidoscopy every 5 years or colonoscopy every 10 years or double contrast barium enema (DCBE) every 5-10 years, with digital rectal examination performed at the time of each screening sigmoidoscopy, colonoscopy, or DCBE
- Fasting glucose testing (every 3 years)
High-Risk Factors *
- Hemoglobin level assessment
- STI testing
- HIV testing
- Tuberculosis skin testing
- Lipid profile assessment
- Thyroid-stimulating hormone testing
- Hepatitis C virus testing
- Colorectal cancer screening

★ *Please see page 10 for High Risk Factors*

EVALUATION AND COUNSELING

Sexuality
- Sexual functioning
- Sexual behaviors
- STIs
    - Partner selection
    - Barrier protection

Fitness and Nutrition
- Dietary/nutrition assessment
- Exercise: discussion of program
- Calcium intake

Psychosocial Evaluation
- Neglect/abuse
- Lifestyle/stress
- Depression/sleep disorders
- Family relationships
- Work/retirement satisfaction

Cardiovascular Risk Factors
- Hypertension
- Dyslipidemia
- Obesity
- Diabetes mellitus
- Sedentary lifestyle

Health/Risk Behaviors
- Hygiene (general and dental)
- Hormone replacement therapy
- Injury prevention
    - Safety belts and helmets
    - Prevention of falls
    - Occupational & Recreational hazards
    - Firearms
- Visual acuity/glaucoma
- Hearing
- Breast self-examination
- Chemoprophylaxis for breast cancer (for high risk women)
- Skin exposure to ultraviolet rays
- Suicide: depressive symptoms
- Tobacco, alcohol, other drug use

IMMUNIZATIONS

Periodic
- Tetanus-diphtheria booster (every 10 yrs)
- Influenza vaccine (annually)
- Pneumococcal vaccine (once)

High-Risk Groups *
- Hepatitis A vaccine
- Hepatitis B vaccine
- Varicella vaccine

Leading Causes of Death:
- Diseases of the heart
- Cancer
- Cerebrovascular diseases
- Chronic obstructive pulmonary diseases
- Pneumonia/influenza
- Diabetes mellitus
- Accidents and adverse effects
- Alzheimer's disease

Leading Causes of Morbidity:
- Arthritis/osteoarthritis
- Back symptoms
- Breast cancer
- Chronic obstructive pulmonary diseases
- Cardiovascular disease
- Deformity or orthopedic impairment
- Degeneration of macula retinae and posterior pole
- Diabetes
- Hearing and vision impairment
- Hypertension
- Hypothyroidism and other thyroid disease
- Influenza
- Nose, throat, and upper respiratory infections
- Osteoporosis
- Skin lesion/dermatoses/dermatitis
- Urinary tract infections
- Urinary tract (other conditions including urinary incontinence)
- Vertigo

* Please see page 10 for High Risk Factors

INTERVENTIONS FOR HIGH-RISK FACTORS

Intervention	High-Risk Factor
• Bacteriuria testing	Diabetes mellitus
• Cholesterol testing	Familial lipid disorders; family history (FH) of premature coronary heart disease; history of coronary heart disease
• Colorectal cancer screening	Colorectal cancer or adenomatous polyps in first-degree relative younger than 60 years or in two or more first-degree relatives of any ages; family history of familial adenomatous polyposis or hereditary nonpolyposis colon cancer; history of colorectal cancer, adenomatous polyps, or inflammatory bowel disease
• Fasting glucose test	Obesity; first-degree relative with diabetes mellitus; member of a high risk ethnic population (eg, African American, Hispanic, Native American, Asian, Pacific Islander); have delivered a baby weighing more than 9 lb or history of gestational diabetes mellitus; hypertensive; high-density lipoprotein cholesterol level of at least 35 mg/dL; triglyceride level of at least 250 mg/dL; history of impaired glucose tolerance or impaired fasting glucose
• Fluoride supplementation	Live in area with inadequate water fluoridation (<0.7 ppm)
• Genetic testing/counseling	Exposure to teratogens; considering pregnancy at age 35 or older; patient partner, or family member with history of genetic disorder or birth defect; African, Eastern European Jewish, Mediterranean, or Italian ancestry
• Hemoglobin level assessment	Caribbean, Latin American, Asian, Mediterranean, or African ancestry; history of excessive menstrual flow
• Hepatitis A vaccination	International travelers; illegal drug users; people who work with nonhuman primates; chronic liver disease; clotting-factor disorders; sex partners of bisexual men; measles, mumps, and rubella nonimmune persons; food-service workers; health-care workers; daycare workers
• Hepatitis B vaccination	Intravenous drug users and their sexual contacts; recipients of clotting factor concentrates; occupational exposure to blood or blood products; patients and workers in dialysis units; persons with chronic renal or hepatic disease; household or sexual contact with hepatitis B virus carriers; history of sexual activity with multiple partners; history of sexual activity with sexually active homosexual or bisexual men; international travelers; residents and staff of institutions for the developmentally disabled and of correctional institutions
• Hepatitis C virus (HCV) testing	History of injecting illegal drugs; recipients of clotting factor concentrates before 1987; chronic (long-term) hemodialysis; persistently abnormal alanine aminotransferase levels; recipient of blood from a donor who later tested positive for HCV infection; recipient of blood or blood-component transfusion or organ transplant before July 1992; occupational percutaneous or mucosal exposure to HCV-positive blood
• Human immunodeficiency virus (HIV) testing	Seeking treatment for STIs; drug use by injection; history of prostitution; past or present sexual partner who is HIV positive or bisexual or injects drugs; long-term residence or birth in an area with high prevalence of HIV infection; history of transfusion from 1978-1985; invasive cervical cancer; pregnancy. Offer to women seeking preconceptional care
• Influenza vaccine	Anyone who wishes to reduce the chance of becoming ill with influenza; resident in long-term care facility; chronic cardiopulmonary disorders; metabolic diseases (e.g., diabetes mellitus, hemoglobinopathies, immunosuppression, renal dysfunction); health-care workers; day-care workers; pregnant women who will be in the second or third trimester during the epidemic season. Pregnant women with medical problems should be offered vaccination before the influenza season regardless of stage of pregnancy
• Lipid profile assessment	Elevated cholesterol level; history of parent or sibling with blood cholesterol of at least 240 mg/dL; first degree relative with premature (<55 years of age for men, <65 years of age for women) coronary artery disease; diabetes mellitus; smoking habit

• Mammography	Women who have had breast cancer or who have a first-degree relative (ie, mother, sister, or daughter) or multiple other relatives who have a history of premenopausal breast or breast and ovarian cancer
• Measles, mumps, rubella vaccine	Adults born in 1957 or later should be offered vaccination (one dose of MMR) if there is no proof or immunity or documentation of a dose given after first birthday; persons vaccinated in 1963-1967 should be offered revaccination (2 doses); health-care workers, students entering college, international travelers, and rubella-negative postpartum patients should be offered a second dose
• Pneumococcal vaccine	Chronic illness such as cardiovascular disease, pulmonary disease, diabetes mellitus, alcoholism, chronic liver disease, cerebrospinal fluid leaks, functional or anatomic asplenia; exposure to an environment where pneumococcal outbreaks have occurred; immunocomprimised patients (eg, HIV infection, hematologic or solid malignancies, chemotherapy, steroid therapy); pregnant patients with chronic illness. Revaccination after 5 years may be appropriate for certain high-risk groups
• Rubella titer assessment	Childbearing age and no evidence of immunity
• STI testing	History of multiple sexual partners or a sexual partner with multiple contacts, sexual contact with persons with culture-proven STI, history of repeated episodes of STIs, attendance at clinics for STIs; routine screening for chlamydial and gonorrheal infection for all sexually active adolescents and other asymptomatic women at high risk for infection
• Skin examination	Increased recreational or occupational exposure to sunlight; family or personal history of skin cancer; clinical evidence of precursor lesions
• Thyroid-stimulating hormone test	Strong family history of thyroid disease; autoimmune disease (evidence of subclinical hypothyroidism may be related to unfavorable lipid profiles)
• Tuberculosis skin test	HIV infection; close contact with persons known or suspected to have TB; medical risk factors known to increase risk of disease if infected; born in country with high TB prevalence; medically underserved; low income; alcoholism; intravenous drug use; resident of long-term care facility (e.g., correctional institutions, mental institutions, nursing homes and facilities); health professional working in high-risk health-care facilities
• Varicella vaccine	All susceptible adults and adolescents, including health-care workers; household contacts of immunocompromised individuals; teachers; day-care workers; residents and staff of institutional settings, colleges, prisons, or military installations; international travellers; non-pregnant women of childbearing age

Advantages of counseling:

- Involves patient in his/her own care and dispels misconceptions, myths and rumors
- Improves success with complicated regimens
- Helps people change risky behaviors— a vital, yet difficult, task
- Facilitates the decision-making process regarding contraception and STI prevention
- Explains possible side effects, which reduces anxiety, increases success with method and encourages clients to return if problems occur, reducing severity of complications
- Builds and strengthens the provider/patient relationship
- Encourages patient responsibility for his/her health decisions
- Ensures and maintains *confidentiality*

Principles of good counseling:

- **Allow plenty of time: so important and so difficult** ◄
- *Listen*, look at your patients, allow them to speak freely, paraphrase what you hear
- Remember LISTEN and SILENT use the same letters!
- *Respect*, recognize and accept each individual's unique situation
- Accept and anticipate that behavior change occurs slowly and incrementally. Remember that *"a lapse is not a relapse" [Prochaska-1994]*
- Remain *sensitive*; acknowledge that sex/sexuality are very personal
- Be *nonjudgmental* and encourage *self-determination*; avoid *false reassurance*
- *Urge all your patients to know their HIV status*; each encounter offers opportunity to counsel about STI/HIV prevention and contraception
- Inquire about problems patients may have had with previous medical recommendations
- Know what you are talking about!
- Realize your patient will remember only 1-4 points. Avoid providing too much information ◄ and provide written information

The GATHER method suggests the following steps:

- **Greet** patient in a warm, friendly manner; help her or him to feel at ease
- **Ask** patient about her or his needs and reproductive goals; ask about risk for STIs
- **Tell** patient about her or his choices, explaining the advantages and disadvantages of all options
- **Help** patient to choose
- **Explain** the correct use of the method or drug being prescribed
- **Repeat** important instructions to the patient and clarify time and conditions of return visit; give written instructions to patient to review later

Reproductive/Contraceptive Goals:

GOAL:	MAIN CONTRACEPTIVE CONCERNS MAY BE:
Delaying birth of first child	Effectiveness of method, future fertility and STIs
Wants to avoid abortion for any reason	Need for maximal effectiveness; Tell about ECs; May want to use 2 methods consistently ◄
Spacing births	Balance of efficacy and convenience
Completed childbearing	Needs effective method for long term: offer IUD, sterilization or other extremely effective methods

Felicia Guest is a remarkable individual and an extremely creative health educator! Here is how she suggested (with credits to Dr. Felicia Stewart) that a girl or woman could decide if a boy or man were a bad or good prospect as a date:

HOW TO PICK A BOYFRIEND:

Don't even think about it! If he...

- Uses drugs or gives you drugs (Rohypnol, Ecstasy)
- Is violent
- Committed a crime

Don't even talk, don't find out his name, just walk away!

You deserve better! Beware if he...

- Is much older
- Has lots of former girlfriends he had sex with
- Doesn't listen to you
- Has children that he is not supporting
- Is having sex currently with another person
- Lies to you
- Uses or wants your money
- Is extremely disrespectful in referring to his mother

This could work! If...

- He respects you
- He has a life plan that fits your life plan
- He listens to you
- He never, ever scares you
- He appeals to you

Sometimes, after hearing the above, a teenager will reply, "but I love him." Felicia Guest suggests the following responses to the "but I love him" remark:
- Love is NOT supposed to hurt

STRUCTURED COUNSELING ◄━━━

Carefully planned structured counseling is very different than counseling.
Structured counseling may involve techniques such as:
• Repetition of a specific message at the time of the initial visit
• Having the patient repeat back her understanding of a message
• Use of a brief, clear, concise videotape
• Asking the patient if she has questions about the videotape
• Written instructions that clearly highlight key messages
• Repetition at each follow-up visit
• Checklist for patient to fill out at ***each*** follow up visit

Discontinuation rates among women started on Depo-Provera are extremely high.
Methodical structured counseling for women starting on Depo-Provera might include:
• **The message: Depo-Provera will change your periods.** No woman's periods stay the same as they were before starting Depo-Provera. Repeating this for the patient at the time of the initial visit and discussion of whether this is acceptable for her
• Having the patient repeat back her understanding of parts of one's message, particularly the message that **over time a woman stops having periods most months** and tends to have very irregular menses almost immediately
• Use of a brief, clear, concise videotape
• Asking the patient if she has questions about the videotape
• Written instructions that clearly highlight the key messages
• Asking at each 3-month visit what has happened to a woman's pattern of bleeding, whether amenorrhea has begun and how she feels about her pattern of bleeding

Checklist for Depo Provera patient to fill out at each follow up visit. Please check yes or no. Tell us if you have:

Spotting or irregular vaginal bleeding	☐ Yes	☐ No
Missed periods or very, very light periods	☐ Yes	☐ No
Concern over your pattern of vaginal bleeding	☐ Yes	☐ No
Depression, severe anxiety or mood changes	☐ Yes	☐ No
Gained 5 pounds or more	☐ Yes	☐ No
Questions you want to ask us about Depo-Provera injections	☐ Yes	☐ No

See STRUCTURED COUNSELING on p. 126 for an analysis of the effect of structured ◄━━━ counseling on Depo-Provera discontinuation rates

Taking Sexual Histories

Although historically health care providers have been reluctant to inquire about sexual issues because of both time and social constraints, more clinicians are realizing that sexual histories are essential to identifying at-risk individuals and to providing appropriate testing and treatment. Explain to the patient that obtaining sexual information is necessary to provide complete care, but reassure her or him that she or he has the right to discuss only what she/he is comfortable divulging. Patients often want correct sex information and need to discuss sexual concerns that may be affecting their sexual performance or satisfaction. Ask patients less direct questions in the beginning to build trust, then ask the questions that explicitly address sexual issues once you have their confidence. Be cautious about what **information** you place on the chart. Charts are not necessarily confidential and can be reviewed by ◄— insurance companies. **Charts may be subpoenaed**

Initiating the Sexual History

- I will be asking some personal questions about your sexual activity to help me make more accurate diagnoses. This is a normal part of the exam I do with all patients
- Is this all right with you? If there are things you do not want me to chart, I won't ◄—
- You only need to tell me as much as you are comfortable sharing
- Some patients have shared concerns with me related to their risks of infections or concerns about particular sexual activities. If you have any concerns, I would be happy to discuss them with you

Sexual History Questions

- **What are you doing to protect yourself from HIV and other infections? OR What are you doing to put yourself at increased risk for AIDS?**
- Do you have questions regarding sex or sexual activity?
- How old were you when you had your first sexual experience?
- Do you have sex with men, women or both?
- Do you think you need contraception? How are you protecting yourself from unwanted pregnancy?
- How many sex partners have you had in the last 3 months? in the last 6 months? in your lifetime?
- How many sex partners does your partner have?
- Do you have penis in vagina sex? penis in mouth sex? or penis in rectum sex?
- Do you drink alcohol or take drugs in association with sexual activity?
- Have you been forced or coerced to have sex?
- Are you currently in a relationship where you feel physically, sexually, or emotionally threatened? ◄—
- As a child, did anyone touch your private body parts or ask you to touch theirs?
- Have you ever had sex for money, food, protection, drugs or shelter?
- Do you enjoy sex? Do you have orgasms? Do you have pain with sex?
- Do you or your partner(s) have any sexual concerns?

Avoid Assumptions: Making assumptions about a patient's sexual behavior and orientation can leave out important information, undermine patient trust and make the patient feel judged or alienated, causing her to withhold information. This can result in diagnostic and treatment errors. Do not assume that patients:

- Are sexually active and need contraception
- Are NOT sexually active (e.g., older patients, young adolescents)
- Are heterosexual, homosexual or bisexual
- Know if their partners have other partners
- Have power (within a relationship) to make or implement their own contraceptive decisions

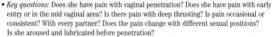

FEMALE

Dyspareunia

- *Definition:* Pain during vaginal intercourse or vaginal penetration
- *Key questions:* Does she have pain with vaginal penetration? Does she have pain with early entry or in the mid vaginal area? Is there pain with deep thrusting? Is pain occasional or consistent? With every partner? Does the pain change with different sexual positions? Is she aroused and lubricated before penetration?
- *Causes:* Organic - vestibulitis, urethritis/UTI, vaginitis, vulvodynia, interstitial cystitis, traumatic deliveries (forcep or vacuum extractions), hypoestrogenism, PID, endometriosis, surgical scars or adhesions, pelvic injuries, tumors, hip joint or disc pain, female circumcision, orgasmic spasm, lack of foreplay, lubrication
  Psychological - current or previous abuse, relationship stress, depression, anxiety, fear of sex
- *Treatment:* Directed to underlying pathology including depression. If dyspareunia is chronic, consider supplementing medical management with supportive counseling and sex therapy

Vaginismus (special case of dyspareunia)

- *Definition:* Painful involuntary spastic contraction of introital and pelvic floor muscles
- *Causes:* Organic - may be secondary to current or previous dyspareunia and its causes.
  Psychological - sexual abuse, fears of abnormal anatomy (e.g. terror that vagina will rip with penile or speculum intercourse), negative attitudes about sexuality
- *Treatment:* Education is critical. Insight into underlying causes helps. After source is recognized, start progressive desensitization exercises, which can include self manipulation and dilators. Sex therapist/psychologist intervention needed to deal with unconscious fears unresponsive to education

Decreased Libido (Hypoactive Sexual Desire)

- *Definition:* Relative lack of sexual desire defined by individual as troublesome to her sexual relationship; there is no absolute "normal" level
- *Causes:* Organic - may be due to acute or chronic debilitating medical condition (e.g., diabetes, stroke, spinal cord injury, arthritis, pain, cancer, chronic obstructive pulmonary disease, coronary artery disease, etc.), medications (e.g. sedatives, narcotics, hypnotics, anticonvulsants, centrally-acting antihypertensives, tranquilizers, anorectics, oral contraceptives, Depo-Provera, and some antidepressants), dyspareunia, incontinence, alcohol, hormonal imbalance, or postpartum healing episiotomy
  Sexual practices - inadequate sexual stimulation or time for arousal. Sexual desires discordant with partner's desires
  Psychological - depression, anxiety, exhaustion, life stress (finances, relationship problems, etc.), poor partner communications, lack of understanding about impacts of aging. Change in body image (breast-feeding, postpartum, weight gain, or post mastectomy or hysterectomy)
- *Treatment:* Treat underlying causes where possible. Rule out hyperactive sexual desire disorder of partner. Reassure about normalcy, if appropriate. Help patient create time and special space for sexual expression - no distractions from children, telephone, household chores. Suggest variety in sexual practices perhaps with aid of fantasies (erotic fiction, films, etc). Physiologic androgen replacement can enhance libido. New drugs, including Viagra and ointments causing increased blood flow to the clitoris, may increase sexual arousal. Consider referral to sex therapist. Read *For Each Other* by Lonnie Barbach and *Women, Sex & Desire* by Elizabeth Davis

Excessive Sexual Desire (Hyperactive Sexual Desire)

- *Definition:* Excessive sexual activity resulting in social, psychological and physical problems.
  See Diagnostic and Statistical Manual of Mental Disorders, Fourth Edition (DSM-IV)
- *Cause:* Low self esteem; abuse at young age; attention seeking; acting out; mania; other
  such as bipolar disease
- *Treatment:* Refer for psychological counseling and therapy, Sex Addicts Anonymous after therapy ◄

Orgasmic Disorders: Anorgasmia or Primary Anorgasmia

- *Definitions:*
  - *Preorgasmia or Primary Anorgasmia:* Never experienced orgasms and desires to be orgasmic
  - *Secondary Anorgasmia:* Orgasmic in past, no orgasms currently, desirous of orgasm
- *Cause:* Organic - may be secondary to dyspareunia, neurological, vascular disease,
  medications (e.g. sedatives, narcotics, hypnotics, anticonvulsants, centrally-acting
  antihypertensives, tranquilizers, anorectics, and some antidepressants - particularly SSRI
  class antidepressants), or poor sexual techniques of partner (painful, rapid ejaculation)
  Psychological - negative attitude about sexuality, chronic relationship stress; lack of
  knowledge about body and sexual response
- *Treatment:* Treat underlying organic causes, if possible. Explain sexual response (suggest
  reading *Our Bodies, Ourselves*). Add behavioral/psychological approach using PLISSIT
  model (see Abbreviations, p. vi), and sensate focusing exercises. Help couple set alternative
  pleasuring goals. Refer to sex therapist if initial interventions not successful. Have woman
  learn how to have an orgasm on her own in comfortable environment and then she can teach
  her partner how to pleasure her. Recommend use of lubricants, vibrators and sex toys. Read ◄
  For Yourself by Lonnie Barbach

MALE

Decreased Libido (Hypoactive sexual desire disorder)

- No absolute level "normal"; "decreased libido" usually related to previous experience,
  partner's expectations
- Evaluation and treatment similar to female's (see above)

Excessive Sexual Desire (Hyperactive Sexual Desire) ◄

- *Definition:* Excessive sexual activity resulting in social, psychological and physical problems.
- *Cause:* Abuse at young age; attention seeking; acting out; mania; other such as bipolar disease
- *Treatment:* Refer for psychological counseling and therapy, Sex Addicts Anonymous after therapy

Premature (Rapid) Ejaculation

- *Definition:* Recurrent ejaculation before or shortly after vaginal penetration or ejaculation
  occurs earlier than patient or partner desires. Average time from entry to ejaculation in
  "normal" couples is 2 minutes; shorter interval is consistent with diagnosis.
- *Causes:* Organic - urethritis, prostatitis, neurological disease (e.g. multiple sclerosis).
  Psychological - learned behavior, result of anxiety (especially among teens)
- *Treatment:* Education and reassurance is important. If goal is pleasuring of partner, teach
  other techniques to arouse her or him prior to intercourse and/or to achieve orgasm.
  "Start and stop" technique can be used to prolong erection; man stops stimulation for at
  least 30 seconds when he feels ejaculation imminent. "Squeeze" technique helpful; when
  man feels impending ejaculation, partner firmly squeezes the head of the penis beneath
  the glans for 4-5 seconds to decrease erection. Selective serotonin reuptake inhibitors
  (SSRIs) in low doses may be helpful if these other techniques are not adequate. Refer to
  sex therapist (or urologist if cause organic) for additional treatment if needed. Durex now
  makes a condom with benzocaine to decrease sensation and help prevent premature ◄
  ejaculation

Delayed (Retarded) Ejaculation/Anorgasmia
- *Definition:* Inability to or difficulty in experiencing orgasm and ejaculation with a partner
- *Cause:* usually psychological; learned behavior; may occur when a man has masturbatory patterns that cannot be duplicated with partner; overemphasis on sexual performance; medications such as SSRI's. Rule out organic problems carefully ◄───
- *Treatment:* referral to sex therapist recommended

Erectile Dysfunction/Disorders (ED) (Impotence)
- *Definition:* Inability to attain or sustain an erection that is satisfactory for coitus
- *Primary:* never achieved erection
  - *Causes:* Organic - low testosterone levels due to hypothalamic-pituitary-testicular disorder; severe vascular compromise. Psychological - usual cause
- *Secondary:* current inability to attain or maintain erection (may be situational)
  - *Causes:* Organic - diabetes mellitus, alcohol abuse, hypothyroidism, drug dependency, medications (e.g. sedatives, narcotics, hypnotics, anticonvulsants, centrally-acting antihypertensives, tranquilizers, anorectics, and some antidepressants), hypopituitarism, penile infections, atherosclerosis, aortic aneurysm, multiple sclerosis, spinal cord lesions, orchiectomy or prostatectomy
  Psychological - depression, relationship stress, prior abuse, etc. Suspect when patient has morning erection or is able to masturbate to ejaculation
- *Treatment:* Treat underlying cause. Switch medications if possible. Same measures that help women's sexual desire may be useful. Medical or mechanical treatments available:
  1. *Testosterone.* Shown to be useful in wasting diseases (AIDS) and other low testosterone conditions. Available in patches for ease of use
  2. *Sildenafil citrate (Viagra)* 25-100 mg (usual dose 50 mg) tablet one hour prior to intercourse. Contraindicated with other ED treatments, retinosis pigmentosa, priapism or nitrates (nitroglycerin, isosorbide mononitrate, isosorbide nitrate, pentaerythritol tetranitrate, erythrityl tetranitrate)
  3. *Alprostadil injections (Edex or Caverject)* prostaglandin E1 ~ 1 cc injected into corpus cavernosa (strengths 125 µg - 1000 µg. Dose determined in office visit.) Excessive injection may cause priapism. Erection achieved with stimulation lasts 30-60 minutes. Avoid in anticoagulated patients and with vasoactive medications. Limit 3 per week
  4. *Alprostadil suppository (Muse)* prostaglandin pellet E1 (125-1000 µg) placed inside urethra. Erection occurs as drug absorbed. 70% successful. Contraindications - anatomical penile abnormalities (strictures, hypospadias, etc.), and thrombosis risk factors. Limit 2/day
  5. *Yohimbine hydrochloride.* Prescription pill composed of indole alkaloid. Modestly successful. Avoid in psychiatric patients (causes agitation and hallucination).
  6. *Vacuum Erection Device (VED).* Use of a vacuum pump and different size rubber bands maintains an erection for 30 minutes. Safe and effective (90% success rate). May be cumbersome and decrease spontaneity
  7. *Penile implants (prostheses).* Permanent bendable rods or inflatable reservoirs implanted surgically into penis. Activated/inflated for intercourse. Success rate high, but associated with surgical risks and the risk that natural erections disappear
  8. *Microsurgery.* Used in men with atherosclerosis of penile arteries or venous pathology; over 50% success rate

---

TO FIND SEX THERAPISTS • Go to www.aasect.org ◄───
  • Call your local Planned Parenthood clinic

Adolescents are very interested in sex, contraception, and STIs, but they rarely raise these issues with their providers. Abstinence is increasing slightly among teens, but most American adolescents have had intercourse before high school graduation. Helping adolescents to grow in self respect, is the most important goal of all who work with teens.

COUNSELING CHALLENGES POSED BY ADOLESCENTS

Teens are not "young adults." Developmentally appropriate approaches are needed
- Age 12-14 – teens are very concrete, egocentric (self-focused) and concerned with personal appearance and acceptance, and have a short attention span
- Age 14-15 – teens are peer oriented and authority resistant (challenge boundaries), and have very limited images of the future
- Age 16-17 – teens are developing logical thought processes and goals for the future

Nonjudgmental, open-ended and reflective questions are better than direct yes-no inquiries. Try reflective questions such as "What would you want to tell a friend who was thinking about having sex?" instead of "You're not having sex, are you?"

CONFIDENTIALITY:
Adolescents are often afraid to obtain medical care for contraception, pregnancy testing or STI treatment because they fear parental reaction. Over two-thirds of teens never discuss with their parents anything sexual that they have done; over one-half feel that their parents could not handle it. All teens should be entitled to confidential services and counseling, but billing systems and/or laws in some states affect their confidential access to family planning services. Know your local laws and refer to sites that may be able to meet all the teen's needs if your practice can not.

ADOLESCENTS AND THE LAW:
This table provides information on an adolescent's right to consent to reproductive health, contraception, and abortion services.

Table 6.1 Adolescents and the Law ◀

AL ●■□★	DC ●■✚	IA ○■✚	MI ○■□★	NH ●■✚	OK ●■□◇	TX ○■□✦
AK ●■☆	FL ●■☆	KS ●■✚	MN ●■□★	NJ ●■◇	OR ●■✚	UT ○■✦
AZ ●■★	GA ●■□✦	KY ○■★	MS ●■★	NM ●■☆	PA ●■★	VT ○■✚
AR ●■□★	HI ●■□✚	LA ○■□★	MO ○■□★	NY ●■✚	RI ○■★	VA ●■✦
CA ●■☆	ID ●■★	ME ●■□✚	MT ●■□◇	NC ●■★	SC ●■★	WA ●■✚
CO ●■✦	IL ●■◇	MD ●■★	NE ○■✦	ND ●■★	SD ●■✦	WV ○■✦
CT ○■✚	IN ○■★	MA ●■★	NV ○■★	OH ○■◇✦	TN ●■★	WI ○■★
DE ●■□✦						WY ●■✦

● = Minor may consent to contraceptive service (including some states with special circumstances such as the minors' health, marital, or pregnancy status)

○ = No explicit policy related to minors' access to contraceptive services

■ = Minor may consent to testing and treatment for STDs

□ = Physician may inform parents about STD testing and treatment but is not required to

★ = Parental consent required before a minor may obtain an abortion

☆ = Parental consent law exists but not in effect (e.g., declared unenforceable by courts)

✦ = Parental notification required before a minor may obtain an abortion. In some states, parental notification is not necessary if a risk for the minor is perceived (i.e. telling parents may result in harm to minor)

◇ = Parental notification law exists but not in effect (e.g., declared unenforceable by courts)

✚ = Does not require parental involvement before a minor may obtain an abortion

Sources: *State Policies in Brief: Parental Involvement in Minors' Abortions; Minors' Access to STD Services; Minors' Access to Contraceptive Services.* As of January 1, 2003. Alan Guttmacher Institute.

Note: Many of the laws contain specific clauses that affect their meaning and application. The authors encourage readers to consult the above documents (updated monthly) for more details: www.agi-usa.org.

PELVIC EXAMS AND BIRTH CONTROL PILLS ◄──

The pelvic exam may be a barrier to a young woman initiating contraceptive services. It is not necessary to perform a pelvic exam prior to prescribing oral contraceptive pills
[Stewart-2001]

ADOLESCENTS AS RISK TAKERS

• Full evaluation of behaviors is important to personalize counseling. Teens must move away from parental authority figures to become independent adult individuals, but, along the way, they may take excessive risks in many areas, including sexuality
• HEADSS interview technique helpful as an organized approach. Ask each teen about Home, Education, Activities, Drugs, Sexuality (activity, orientation and abuse) and Suicide
• Guidelines for Adolescent Preventive Services (GAPS) developed to help health care providers encourage adolescents to prevent or modify health-compromising behaviors
• Look for the female athletic triad: eating disorders, amenorrhea and osteoporosis. ◄── This triad of symptoms may also occur in women who do not exercise excessively

SEX EDUCATION

The sex education, contraception and STIs curricula offered in many schools sometimes are not medically correct and only covered superficially. Information teens obtain from peers is also often inaccurate, common myths are:
• *You cannot get pregnant the first time you have intercourse*
• *You cannot get pregnant if you douche after sex*
• *Having a baby makes you a woman, makes your boyfriend love you, and gets you the attention you deserve*
• *Making a girl pregnant means that you are a man*

Adolescents need very concrete information and opportunities to role play and practice:
• How to open and place a condom and where to carry it
• How to negotiate NOT having sex
• How to negotiate condom use with sex partner
• How to punch out the pills, where to keep the pack, and how to remember them ◄──
• How to move in direction of dual protection: condoms and another contraceptive
• How to remember when to return for Depo-Provera injections
• How to use emergency contraception, the patch and the vaginal ring ◄──
• How to take oral contraceptives continuously ◄──

ADOLESCENT HEALTH RESOURCES
American Medical Association: (800) 621-8335

AMA Guidelines for Adolescent Preventive Services (GAPS): Recommendations and Rationale
Internet

• Adolescent Health On-Line: www.ama-assn.org/adolhlth/adolhlth.htm
• Division of Adolescent and School Health, National Center for Chronic Disease Prevention and Health Promotion, Centers for Disease Control and Prevention: www.cdc.gov/nccdphp/dash/index.htm
• Society for Adolescent Medicine: www.adolescenthealth.org

PERIMENOPAUSE: The 3-5 years toward the end of the reproductive life of a woman when her ovarian follicles are less responsive to stimulation. An important marker of the perimenopause is menstrual irregularity. Fluctuations in ovarian hormonal production can result in intermittent vasomotor symptoms, menstrual disturbances and reduced fertility. It is important to remember, though, that even with reduced fertility, a perimenopausal woman needs contraception until she is truly menopausal (no menses x 1 yr). Perimenopausal women have the highest abortion rate (# abortions/ # pregnancies) of any group except women under 15

- All methods of birth control are available to eligible women until menopause
- In the United States, 50% of all contracepting women age 40-44 have been sterilized and another 20% have a partner with a vasectomy
- Oral contraceptive pills, patches, rings, hormonal IUDs, or combined injections may ◄— provide the additional benefits of control of DUB, prevention of osteoporosis, hot flashes and irregular cycles. Benefits of the Mirena IUD for women with menorrhagia are remarkable (see p. 87). Estrogen-containing contraceptives should not be used in women over 35 ◄— who smoke. Smokers may use POPs or DMPA, IUDs, or barriers.

Health Screening: see Chapter 2 for screening guidelines by age

MENOPAUSE: The permanent cessation of spontaneous menses, at an average age 51-52, creates an excellent opportunity to encourage healthy diets, exercise and health-promoting lifestyles (smoking cessation, calcium supplementation, etc.). Perhaps the single most important lifestyle message is that women who smoke as little as 1-4 cigarettes/day have a 2.5 fold increased risk of fatal coronary artery disease *[Speroff · 1999, p. 649]*

Common Physiologic Changes After Estrogen Loss

- Hot flashes/sleep disturbances, mood swings, decreased ability to concentrate and remember
- Thinning of genital urinary tissue (atrophic vaginitis, urinary incontinence)
- Osteopenia, osteoporosis, increased risk for fracture
- Increased risk for cardiovascular disease, unfavorable lipid profiles, increased vascular resistance, increased homocysteine levels
- Increased risk for colon cancer
- Other possible consequences of estrogen deficiency: increased risk of Alzheimer's disease, colon cancer, tooth loss, macular degenerative eye disease, decreased collagen and ◄— skin wrinkling, decreased short-term memory

HORMONE REPLACEMENT THERAPY (HRT, HT or ERT): A woman may choose ERT or HRT for short-term indications and then revisit that decision at a later date. Each woman should be informed of potential benefits and risks of hormone replacement therapy individualized to her own situation as part of a comprehensive health promotion program which also emphasizes proper nutrition and exercise. HRT is therapeutic in relieving vasomotor symptoms (hot flashes, night sweats) but is also used as preventive therapy to reduce some of the long term sequelae of estrogen deficiency: increased risk of vertebral, radial and femoral head fracture, and genital atrophy. 60% of females between the ages of 55-64 are sexually active. HRT (estrogen component) helps alleviate decreased lubrication and genital atrophy. The results of the widely publicized ◄— Women's Health Initiative study on combination HRT *[Writing Group WHI-2002]* have changed the landscape of prescribing HRT. Specifically, the conclusion of the articles states "Results from WHI indicate that the combined postmenopausal hormones CEE, 0.625 mg/d, plus MPA, 2.5 mg/d should not be initiated or continued for the primary prevention of CHD. In addition, the substantial risks for cardiovascular disease and breast cancer must be weighed against the benefit for reduction in fracture risk, reduction in colorectal cancer risk, relief of menopausal symptoms in selecting from the available agents." This randomized trial quantifies these risks that women taking conjugated equine estrogen (CEE 0.625)/MPA 2.5 mg face: invasive breast cancer 1.26, coronary heart disease 1.29, stroke 1.41 and pulmonary embolism

PRESCRIBING PRECAUTIONS FOR HRT

- Pregnancy; undiagnosed abnormal vaginal bleeding
- Active liver disease
- Recent or active thrombophlebitis or thromboembolic disorders (unless anticoagulated)
- Breast cancer or known or suspected estrogen-dependent neoplasm
- Recent myocardial infarction or severe cardiac artery disease

STARTING HRT

- Patient counseling is key to success with HRT. Clearly describe onset of action of HRT for women with hot flashes as well as side effects (especially vaginal spotting and bleeding)
- Answer all questions about risks including a slightly increased risk for breast cancer, deep vein thrombosis, pulmonary embolism and cardiovascular disease *[WHI-2002]* ◄──
- Recent routine history and physical examination sufficient to identify any contraindications.
- Usual well-women care measures (e.g. mammogram, pap smear, lipid profile, thyroid function tests) should be provided but are not essential prior to starting HRT. Endometrial biopsy not needed except when evaluating abnormal vaginal bleeding
- Women who have had oophorectomy or older women may need androgen supplementation
- Re-evaluate need for HRT/ERT annually. The current HRT products are: ◄──

Generic names - Estrogens	Brand names
Conjugated estrogen tablets, USP	Premarin®
Synthetic conjugated estrogens, A tablets	Cenestin®
Esterified estrogens tablets	Estratab®, Menest®
Estropipate tablets	Ogen®, Ortho-est®
Estradiol tablets	Estrace®
Matrix estradiol transdermal systems	Alora®, Climara®, FemPatch®, Vivelle™, Esclim
Reservoir estradiol transdermal systems	Estraderm®

Generic names - Progestins *	Brand names
Medroxyprogesterone acetate (MPA) tablets	Amen®, Curretab®, Cycrin®, Provera®
Megestrol acetate tablets	Megace®
Norethindrone tablets	Micronor®, Nor-QD®, Norlutin®
Norethindrone acetate tablets	Aygestin®
Micronized progesterone capsules	Prometrium®
Progesterone vaginal gel	Crinone®

*In addition, insertion of Mirena, the levonorgestrel IUD ◄──

Generic names - Combined Products	Brand names
Estradiol and norgestimate tablets	Prefest®
Conjugated estrogens and MPA tablets	Premphase®, Prempro®
Esterified estrogens and methyl testosterone tablets	Estratest®, Estratest® H.S.
Ethinyl estradiol and norethindrone acetate tablets	Femhrt®
Estradiol and norethindrone acetate tablets	Activella™
Matrix estradiol/ norethindrone acetate transdermal systems	CombiPatch™

FOLLOW-UP

- Be available to answer questions when there are media reports about HRT
- Patient should return in 1-3 months to answer further questions/manage side effects
- Have the woman keep a menstrual calendar of any breakthrough bleeding or spotting
- If hot flashes continue, consider thyroid dysfunction and other causes before increasing dose or using other therapeutic approaches to hotflash treatment

At least one month before pregnancy, women should start taking folic acid supplements. Folic acid should be taken by all women at risk for pregnancy i.e. by most women in the reproductive years.

Assess:

- Reproductive, family and personal medical and surgical history with attention to pelvic surgeries
- Smoking, drug use, alcohol use: advise to stop and refer for help if needed
- Nutrition habits: identify excesses and inadequacies
- Medications: make adjustments in those that may affect fertility and/or pregnancy outcome. Advise patient not to make any changes without clinician's knowledge
- Risk for sexually transmitted infection/infertility
- Impacts of any medications (over-the-counter, prescription, herbal). For example, Accutane and tetracycline(which are teratogenic) for acne requires extremely effective contraception and strong consideration of the use of 2 contraceptives correctly and consistently. For Accutane repeated negative pregnancy tests are necessary. Accutane can cause severe congenital anomalies in a developing fetus. Advise Accutane patients to delay pregnancy for 1 month after last dose. See p. 37 ←

Offer Screening for:

- Infections (TB, gonorrhea, chlamydia, HIV, syphilis, hepatitis B & C, as per CDC guidelines). Vaginal wet mount if discharge present
- Neoplasms (breast, cervical dysplasia, warts, etc.)
- Immunity (rubella, tetanus, chicken pox, HBV)

Provide Genetic Counseling:

- Advanced maternal age
- Previous poor pregnancy outcomes
- Family history of mental retardation or genetic disorders
- Sickle cell anemia, thalassemia, cystic fibrosis, Tay-Sachs, Canavan disease
- High risk ethnic backgrounds - African Americans, Ashkenazi Jews, etc.
- Alcohol use, tobacco use, substance abuse
- Seizure disorders
- Diabetes, neural tube defects
- Other heritable medical problems

Assess Environmental Hazards:

- Chemical, radioactive and infectious exposures at workplace, home, hobbies
- Physical conditions, especially workplace

Assess Psychosocial Factors:

- Readiness of woman and partner for parenthood
- Mental health (depression, etc.) and domestic violence
- Financial issues and support systems

Recommend:

- *Ideally, planning a pregnancy should involve both a woman and her partner*
- Balanced diet
- Limit fish from local waters to 6 oz/week. Other fish (swordfish, etc) to 12 oz/week (ACOG, EPA)
- Prenatal vitamin with 0.4 mg folic acid for all women (use higher dose folic acid, 4 mg, in higher-risk women such as women with previous neural tube defect, diet with minimal vegetable intake, alcoholic, malabsorption or on anticonvulsants)
- Minimize STI exposure risk
- Weight loss, if obese (gradual loss until conception)
- Moderate exercise
- Avoiding exposure to cat feces (toxoplasmosis) ←
- Early in process of discussing pregnancy encourage breastfeeding as the best way to ← feed her baby

Avoid

- Raw meat (including fish) and unpasteurized dairy products
- Abdominal/pelvic X-rays, if possible
- Excesses in diet, vitamins, exercise
- Non-foods (pica), unusual herbs
- Sex with multiple partners or sex with a partner who may be HIV-positive, have other STI or have other sex partner(s). Use condom if any question

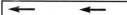

Here's a tip for people who have used this book in the past: in one or two hours you can find the major changes in the 2003-2004 edition. Simply thumb through the pages looking for the arrows! This would also be an excellent way to give a lecture on "what's new in family planning."

Early testing gives a woman a head start to pursue pregnancy options
- Prenatal care can be initiated promptly
- Ectopic pregnancies may be detected earlier
- If she desires abortion, can have choice of medical or surgical method, in part depending on gestational age

PREGNANCY TESTS

Urine tests:
- *Enzyme-linked immunosorbent assay (ELISA) test:*
  - Immunometric test uses antibody specific to placentally-produced HCG and another antibody to produce a color change. Commonly used in home pregnancy test and in offices and clinics
  - Performed in 1-3 minutes using urine samples
  - Test turns positive at levels of 25 mIU/ml. This level can be detectable 7-10 days after conception. May require 5-7 days after implantation to detect all pregnancies
  - Urine pregnancy tests are used in most clinical settings and are available for women to purchase in drugstores; teach patients that no lab test is 100% accurate and that false negative tests (tests read as negative when a woman actually is pregnant) usually occur when done too early in the pregnancy and are far more common than false positive tests (tests read as positive when a woman actually is NOT pregnant)

Serum tests (blood drawn):
- *Radioimmunoassay:*
  - Uses colorimetry, which detects HCG levels as low as 5 mIU/ml
  - Results available in 1-2 hours
  - Offers ability to quantify levels of HCG to monitor levels over time when clinically indicated

HCG QUICK FACTS
- β-HCG can be detected as early as 7-10 days after conception thereby, "ruling in" pregnancy, but pregnancy cannot be "ruled out" until 7 days after expected menses
- A sensitive (urine or serum) pregnancy test can be positive 1-2 days after implantation
- In a normal pregnancy, serum HCG values double every 1.5 days before 5 weeks gestation and every 2 days between 5-7 weeks
- If needed for evaluation of early pregnancy, serial HCG testing should be done every 2 days until levels reach discriminatory levels of 1800-2000 mIU/ml, when a gestational sac can be visualized reliably by vaginal ultrasound. Normally the level doubles every 48 hours
- Average time for HCG levels to become non-detectable after first trimester abortion (medical or surgical) ranges from 31-38 days

MANAGEMENT TIPS
- Home tests can be misused or misinterpreted.
- Any test can have false-negative results at low levels. If in doubt, repeat urine test in 1-2 days or obtain serum tests with a qualitative HCG radioimmunoassay

PREGNANCY TEST NEGATIVE: A TEACHABLE MOMENT

A negative pregnancy test for a woman *not* wanting to become pregnant clearly provides
the counselor or clinician with a teachable moment and a time to offer a woman ECPs ◄—
for future acts of intercourse that might be unprotected.

"Phew! The pregnancy test is negative." This must have been scary to worry that you
might be pregnant.

1. If you haven't been using contraception, this is your "wake-up call." What
   contraceptive method would work best for you now?
2. Abstinence may be your chosen path now; if not, use contraception unless you want
   to become pregnant. Give her contraception now. Don't make her wait for another
   appointment. We can give most contraceptives without a pelvic exam.
3. Learn about emergency contraceptive pills and emergency IUD insertion.
4. Don't try to become pregnant in order to see if you can become pregnant.
5. Take the path less traveled sexually. Don't take a chance from this moment on:
   never, just never, have intercourse without knowing that you are protected against
   both infection and unintended or unwanted pregnancy.
6. Remember, your negative urine pregnancy test does not rule out conception from
   acts of intercourse in the past 2 weeks.
7. Provide emergency contraceptive pills (advance provision works).

PREGNANCY TEST POSITIVE: A TEACHABLE MOMENT

The pregnancy test is positive and she wants to continue the pregnancy. Whether or not this
pregnancy was planned,* your patient's mind is made up: she will continue this pregnancy,
providing you, the counselor or clinician, with a teachable moment.

The pregnancy test is positive and she has definitely decided to continue her pregnancy to term

1. Start folic acid (0.4 mg) in prenatal vitamins today. Buy some prenatal vitamins on
   the way home. ALL WOMEN IN REPRODUCTIVE YEARS SHOULD BE ON FOLIC ACID
2. Stop drinking alcohol today.
3. Stop smoking today.
4. Find the person who will follow you during your pregnancy and tell your health care
   provider if you are on any medication.
5. Use condoms if at any risk for HIV or other STIs.
6. Eat healthy foods. Gain 25-30 pounds during your pregnancy (if your weight is now
   normal).

* If she doesn't want to continue pregnancy, discuss pregnancy termination options
or refer her to someone else who would feel comfortable doing this. Also discuss giving
baby up for adoption

—► 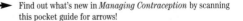 Find out what's new in *Managing Contraception* by scanning
this pocket guide for arrows!

Planning for postpartum contraception should begin during pregnancy and use should be initiated as early as possible postpartum. A newborn can place many demands on a woman's time, so her method should be as convenient for her to use as possible. In some women who are not consistently breastfeeding, ovulation may return within 3-6 weeks postpartum (before a woman realizes she is at risk). Some PP women will choose to return to the use of abstinence as their contraceptive.

AT DELIVERY
- Tubal sterilization may be performed (at C-section or after vaginal delivery)
- IUD may be inserted within 20 minutes of delivery of placenta (requires special equipment/training)

PRIOR TO LEAVING HOSPITAL
- Breastfeeding should be encouraged. Reinforce education about lactational amenorrhea if patient interested (see Chapter 15, p. 40-45)
- Pelvic rest (no douching, no sex, no tampons) is generally recommended for 4-6 weeks. Many women choose NOT to follow this advice in spite of increased risk for infection. Some clinicians encourage women to become sexually active when they feel comfortable and ready
- Women are strongly advised to abstain from intercourse until lochia has stopped.
  Contraception should be selected and provided before patient leaves hospital. Options:
  - Tubal sterilization
  - Progestin-only methods: implants, Depo-Provera (DMPA), progestin-only (mini) pills (POPs)
    NOTE: There are three approaches to starting these progestin-only methods: 1) When the patient leaves the hospital have her start oral iron if her hemoglobin is low and start POPs or DMPA; 2) Since progestin-only methods may prolong bleeding wait 2-3 weeks to start them (no data). Women with history of or high risk for postpartum depression may also benefit from a delay in starting progestin-only methods; 3) In breastfeeding women wait until 6 wks because of concerns, entirely theoretical, that the neonate may be at risk of exposure to hormones in the first 6 weeks. However, since progestin only methods may be the most effective method for a woman, delay in providing these methods on the basis of a purely theoretical concern is not recommended by many clinicians and programs.
  - Male or female condoms to reduce risk of pelvic infection
  - Estrogen containing contraceptive may be prescribed for nonlactating to start 3-4 weeks postpartum (risk of thrombosis associated with pregnancy reduced by that time)
  - IUD may be inserted

AT POSTPARTUM VISIT (3-6 WEEKS)
- Ask if woman has resumed sexual intercourse ◄—
- Encourage breastfeeding
- Lactational amenorrhea follow-up. Provide condoms as transitional method prn return of menses, decrease in breastfeeding, etc
- Emergency contraception may be given if needed. PLAN B is most effective ECP
- Progestin-only methods may be provided (Norplant, Depo-Provera, progestin-only pills). Provide back-up method as needed if initiated when not on menses
- COCs, patch, ring or combined injectables may be started unless woman is exclusively breastfeeding. Provide backup method as needed
- IUD may be inserted if uterus well involuted (whether or not she is breast-feeding)
- Condoms (male or female) may be given as primary or backup contraceptive to provide STI risk reduction; withdrawal can be used at any time
- Tubal sterilization may be provided after uterine involution
- Diaphragm/cervical cap may be fitted after pelvis/cervix return to normal configuration
- NFP and FAM should await resumption of normal cycles

27

CHAPTER 11

Elective Abortion

www.prochoice.org/naf or www.earlyoptionpill.com

OVERVIEW

The availability of safe elective abortion procedures is important for fertility control; 48% of pregnancies in this country are unintended.

Surgical abortion techniques (especially uterine aspiration) have a proven safety profile, with serious morbidity in less than 1% of procedures and a death rate of 0.5/100,000 abortions (compared to maternal mortality with a continued pregnancy of approximately 7.3/100,000 deliveries). The introduction of several agents for early medical abortion have added new options.

Despite having one of the highest abortion rates among developed countries, in 1995 over 78% of US counties had no abortion providers or facilities. It is now up to 86%. Many state laws impose mandatory restrictions, waiting periods, and consent requirements. For current information on your state's abortion laws, contact National Abortion Rights Action League (NARAL)(changing name to Pro Choice America) (202-973-3000 or www.naral.org/) for a copy of "A State-By-State Review of Abortion and Reproductive Rights." Approximately 1.2 million abortions are performed in the U.S. each year; 88% are first trimester and 97% are surgical.

The pattern of induced abortions in the United States has changed from 1994 to 2000:

- The likelihood of a reproductive age woman having an abortion fell 11%
- Abortions among 15-17 year old women fell 39%
- Abortions among 18-19 year olds fell 18%
- Abortions for women at less than 100% above poverty increased 25%
- Abortions for women at 100-199% above poverty level increased 23%
- In 2000, 25% of all pregnancies ended in an induced abortion. *[Jones-2002]*

Features of Medical Compared to Surgical Abortion

Medical	Surgical
Generally avoids invasive procedure	Involves invasive procedure
Requires multiple visits	Usually requires one visit
Days to weeks until complete	Usually complete in a predictable period of time
Available during very early pregnancy	Available during early and later pregnancy
High success rate (95% - 98%)	High success rate (99%)
Requires follow-up to ensure completion of abortion	Does not require follow-up in all cases
May be more private in some circumstances; will vary for each individual patient	May be more private in some circumstances; will vary for each individual patient
Patient participation in multi-step process	Less patient participation in a single-step process
	Allows use of sedation or anesthesia if desired

ELECTIVE SURGICAL ABORTION

DESCRIPTION

Voluntary termination of pregnancy using uterine aspiration in early intrauterine gestations. In later gestations (after 14 weeks) use instruments for tissue removal (dilation and extraction, D & E).

EFFECTIVENESS

- 98-99% effective; failures are mostly incomplete abortions with small amounts of retained tissue; rarely does the pregnancy continue

PROCEDURE

- After informed consent obtained according to local law, type of procedure is determined by gestational age and patient preference
- May dilate the cervix with an osmotic mechanical dilator such as laminaria if > 12 weeks or with a prostaglandin analogue such as misoprostol with or without laminaria in second trimester
- Antibiotic prophylaxis may reduce risk of post-procedure infection.
  Doxycycline 200 mg 30-60 minutes prior to or immediately after procedure or metronidazole 1 g preoperatively and 500 mg orally every 6 hours for 3 doses.
  In areas of high chlamydia prevalence, a 7-day course of doxycycline, or a single dose of azithromycin 1 g may be given preoperatively
- Cleanse ectocervix and endocervix
- Administer cervical anesthesia; if desired, adjunctive sedation can also be used. NSAIDS are administered by some clinicians. Adding a small dose of vasopressin (1-5 units) to cervical anesthetic may reduce risk of hematometra in first trimester abortion and significantly reduces blood loss in second trimester abortions
- Place tenaculum and mechanically dilate cervix if not previously dilated adequately
- Using sterile technique, insert a plastic cannule and apply suction to aspirate products of conception either with a machine, or manually with a syringe (in MVA-manual vacuum aspiration)
- May confirm adequacy of procedure by checking uterine cavity with a sharp curette (optional)
- Evaluate tissue to confirm presence of placental villi/gestational sac if early pregnancy. If more than 9 weeks should be able to visualize fetal tissue
- Administer Rh immune globulin if woman is Rh negative

ADVANTAGES

- Provides woman complete control over her fertility
- Ability to prevent an unwanted or defective birth or halt a pregnancy that poses risk to maternal health or other aspects of her life that she deems important
- Safe and rapid; preoperative evaluation and procedure can usually be done in a single visit from a medical perspective (local legal restrictions may affect this)
- No increase in risk of breast cancer, infertility, cervical incompetence, preterm labor, or congenital anomalies in subsequent pregnancy after uncomplicated first-trimester abortion
- Safer for maternal health than continuing pregnancy
- Can be provided as early as intrauterine pregnancy is diagnosed

DISADVANTAGES

- Most women experience cramping and pain with procedure; the noise of the vacuum machine (if electrical vacuum used) may cause anxiety. (Manual vacuum aspiration or MVA may be more tolerable for this reason) ◄
- Possibility of later regret (regret is equally possible for undesired pregnancy that is continued)

COMPLICATIONS

- Infection <1%
- Incomplete abortion 0.5%-1.0%; Failed abortion 0.1%-0.5%
- Hemorrhage 0.03%-1.0%
- Post-abortal syndrome (hematometra) <1%
- Asherman's syndrome rare (usually in setting of septic abortion)
- Infertility an uncommon complication, related to PID or Asherman's syndrome
- Mortality: Elective abortion deaths <1 per 100,000 (compared to pregnancy deaths/childbirth 7.3/100,000) (Safer than pregnancy or tonsilectomy)

CANDIDATES FOR USE

- Any woman requesting abortion. State laws often limit gestational age (typically available through 24 weeks). State laws may also affect access and consent procedures
- *Adolescents:* State laws vary regarding requirements and consent requirements (See p. 19)

INITIATING METHOD

- Carefully discuss all pregnancy options, including prenatal care for parenting or for adoption and programs available for assistance with each option
- If patient chooses abortion, discuss available techniques when applicable (surgical versus medical)
- Obtain informed consent after answering all questions
- Offer emotional support, education, pre- and post-procedural instructions, and contraception
- Usually perform procedure in outpatient setting unless woman has severe medical problems requiring more intense monitoring or deeper anesthesia

INSTRUCTIONS

- Keep telephone number(s) nearby for any emergencies
- May resume usual activities same day if procedure done under local anesthesia
- One week pelvic rest (no tampons, douching or sexual intercourse)
- Use NSAIDs or acetaminophen for cramping, NSAIDs or ergometrin (methergine) for bleeding
- Showers, baths and swimming are permitted
- Seek medical care urgently if heavy bleeding, excessive cramping, pain, fevers, chills, or malodorous discharge
- Use contraception with every single act of intercourse and keep EC available for future use

FOLLOW-UP

- Have you had a temperature >100.4°F
- What has your bleeding been like since the procedure?
- Have you had any new abdominal or pelvic pain?
- Do you plan to have children? OR Do you plan to have more children?
- Are you using a contraceptive? ◄

PROBLEM MANAGEMENT

Infection
- Always evaluate possibility of retained products and need for reaspiration
- Patients who develop endometritis can generally be treated using outpatient PID therapies described in the CDC Guidelines (see Chapter 31 p. 161)
- Cases that are more complicated may require hospitalization and intravenous antibiotics

Persistent or excessive bleeding
- *Uterine atony* - Rule out retained products and infection. Use uterine-contracting agents (prostaglandin analogues) such as hemabate 250 mcg IM or misoprostol 400-800 mcg rectally (prostaglandin analogue)or vascular constricting agents (methergine) ◄
- *Cervical laceration* - Suture external tears if bleeding significantly, tamponade endocervical lacerations with inflated Foley balloon or similar device or clamp area
- *Retained products of conception* - Reaspiration and consider antibiotics
- *Uterine perforation* - Observe closely; evaluate surgically if any concern about bowel perforation or vascular injury; give antibiotics
- *Hemorrhage* - transfuse to replace large blood loss; provide blood factors to patients with coagulopathies. In rare cases, may need to provide uterine tamponade while transporting to center for further treatment (e.g. embolization, hysterectomy, etc.)

Post-abortal syndrome
- Hematometra (intrauterine clots after procedure). Painful. Blood may not be visible vaginally. Most common at 11-14 weeks (gestational age). Treat with repeat suction curettage and methergine (.2 mg) for 1-3 days. Adding small doses of vasopressin (1-5 units added) to cervical anesthesia at time of initial procedure may reduce risk

Failed abortion
- Can be due to uterine anomaly, twin gestation, or ectopic pregnancy. Obtain ultrasound. Repeat procedure if indicated

Incomplete abortion/retained products of conception
- Reaspirate

FERTILITY AFTER USE
- Immediate return to baseline fertility. Contraceptive should be supplied immediately
- All methods may be initiated the day of a first or second trimester abortion

ELECTIVE MEDICAL ABORTION WITH MIFEPRISTONE (RU-486) (MIFEPREX) AND MISOPROSTOL (MIS)

DESCRIPTION
- Mifepristone (200-600 mg) is administered first and acts as antiprogesterone to block continued support of pregnancy; 600 mg is FDA approved dose - but 200 mg is just as ◄ effective in clinical trials
- Misoprostol is typically given 24 hours later to induce expulsion of the products of ◄ conception
- Used as abortifacient in France since 1988 and in other European countries and China. With some regimens, using misoprostol 800 micrograms vaginally, can be used up to 63 days gestation

EFFECTIVENESS
- Mifepristone followed by MIS 92-98% effective depending on gestational age and MIS doses used

MECHANISMS

- Mifepristone blocks progesterone receptors and inhibits transcription, resulting in down-regulation of progesterone-dependent genes. This causes decidual necrosis and detachment of products of conception. Mifepristone also causes cervical softening
- Misoprostol induces uterine contractions and cervical softening and expulsion of pregnancy (may be taken orally or vaginally either in the office or at home) ◄

ADVANTAGES

- Can be more effective with certain regimens and generally is more rapid
- Can be used up to 63 days gestational age if misoprostol (800 mcg) given vaginally. FDA guidelines state 49 days ◄
- Very early abortions can be performed ◄
- Potentially private method ◄
- Less risk of operative complications ◄
- Some women feel more in control of procedure, feel it is more "natural" ◄
- Provides option to women who may not have access to surgical options, but women need access to surgical care in case D & C is needed ◄

DISADVANTAGES: *Similar to methotrexate except*

- Not effective for ectopics. Need to confirm IUP before administering regimen ◄
- Result not usually delayed
- May need to provide prolonged access to bathroom facilities if patients observed in office after misoprostol administration

COMPLICATIONS *[Silvestre, 1990]*

- Incomplete abortion (2%)
- Ongoing pregnancy (1%) (with exposure to potential teratogen) ◄
- Hemorrhage requiring emergency curettage (<1%)
- Blood transfusion (0.1%)
- Infection (0.1%)

CANDIDATES FOR USE: *Similar to methotrexate candidates (p. 33) except:*

- Gestational age up to 49 days if using oral misoprostol (confirmed intrauterine pregnancy) ◄
- Gestational age up to 63 days if using vaginal misoprostol (confirmed intrauterine pregnancy) ◄
- Not for use by chronic corticosteroid users, chronic adrenal failure, porphyrias, or with history of allergy to methotrexate or prostaglandins

Adolescents: A small study of mifepristone abortion in minors demonstrated high rates of overall acceptability, 75% at day 4-8 and 96% at 4 weeks. At the 4-8 day visit, 82% of participants said they "would choose this procedure over a surgical abortion," compared to 96% at 4 weeks. Cramping pain was deemed acceptable by 36% at day 4-8 and by 71% at 4 weeks *[Phelps, 2001]*

INITIATING METHOD: *Similar to methotrexate (p. 33) except for protocol:*

- **Day 1:** Mifepristone 200-600 mg orally (Mifeprex). Rh immunoglobulin if Rh negative
- **Day 2 or 3:** Give misoprostol (800 µg into posterior fornix of vagina or 400 µg orally) ◄ May observe patient 4 hrs; 44-70% of abortions occur in this time. Most Planned Parenthood clinics are now having patients place this at home with telephone follow-up
- **Day 15:** Assess expulsion; pelvic exam, ultrasound (if needed). For an incomplete or failed abortion, perform D&C or offer observation or repeat misoprostol if only tissue ◄ present (not fetus) and return appointment in 2-4 weeks

INSTRUCTIONS FOR PATIENT, PROBLEM MANAGEMENT, & FERTILITY AFTER USE

- Similar to methotrexate (p. 33)

ELECTIVE MEDICAL ABORTION WITH METHOTREXATE & MISOPROSTOL

DESCRIPTION
Combination medical agents:
- Methotrexate (MTX) is administered first to prevent continued implantation of the pregnancy. Dose: 50 mg/m² IM OR 50 mg PO ◄
- Misoprostol (MIS) is given 3-7 days later to induce expulsion of the products of conception

EFFECTIVENESS
- Complete abortion rate 95% up to 49 days gestation (rates drop to 84% if 50-56 days)
- Like surgical abortion, most failures are incomplete abortions; continuing pregnancy is rare
- 12-35% of women have 20-30 day delay in abortion

MECHANISMS
- MTX prevents reduction of folic acid to tetrahydrofolate by binding to dihydrofolate reductase. This prevents proliferation of placental villi by interfering with DNA synthesis
- The addition of MIS increases uterine contractions to expel the products of conception

ADVANTAGES
- Provides a woman with reproductive choice (see ELECTIVE SURGICAL ABORTION, p. 29-31)
- Very early abortions can be performed; potentially private method
- Therapeutic for ectopic pregnancy in 90-95% of cases
- Less risk of operative complications (risk present only if aspiration required)
- Some women feel more in control of procedure, feel it is more "natural"
- Provides option to women who may not have access to surgical options (although need to have provider available to perform suction curettage if required)

DISADVANTAGES: Now, for the most part, replaced by mifepristone ◄
- Cramping, abdominal pain, nausea (3-66%), vomiting (2-25%), diarrhea (3-52%), fever and chills (8-60%). 40-90% of women take pain reliever
- Vaginal bleeding averages 10-17 days
- May be up to 1 month delay before abortion is complete
- Methotrexate (MTX) and misoprostol (MIS) are Class X drugs (teratogens); follow-up is essential to ensure that the abortion is complete

COMPLICATIONS
- Failed abortion (continuing pregnancy with exposure to Class X teratogen)
- Incomplete abortion
- Approximately 5% will require surgical abortion
- Hemorrhage (women may experience blood clots as may some women during a normal menstrual period)
- Infection, neutropenia, stomatitis or oral ulcers (< 1%)

CANDIDATES FOR USE
- Pregnant women, gestational age ≤ 49 days (well dated by LMP and/or ultrasound) desiring medical termination of pregnancy
- Women willing to abstain from sexual intercourse, alcohol and folate supplements until procedure complete and to comply with visit schedule
- Women who are not anemic or have coagulation disorders, are on anticoagulants, or ◄ have kidney or liver dysfunction

INITIATING METHOD

- Carefully discuss all pregnancy options, including prenatal care for parenting or for adoption and highlight programs available for assistance with each option
- If patient chooses elective abortion, discuss available techniques (surgical vs. medical)
- Review protocol, risks, benefits and visit schedule
- Assess patient's access to provider if D&C is needed. Explain need for D&C if ◄─── incomplete or ongoing (some women think they can avoid surgery altogether)
- Obtain informed consent after all questions are answered

Protocol (adapted from National Abortion Federation Guidelines):

Day 1: Baseline labs including blood type with Rh, hemoglobin (liver function tests and creatinine, if clinically indicated); gestational age ≤ 49 days. Vaginal ultrasound to confirm dates if available. Administer MTX 50 mg/m^2 body surface area IM or 50 mg orally

Day 3-7: MIS 800 µg. Patient self-inserts tablets into posterior fornix of vagina (usually 4 x 200 mg tabs - some clinicians have found them more effective when each tablet is moistened with saline or water). Administer Rh immunoglobulin, if Rh negative

Day 8: Ultrasound; if sac present, repeat dose of MIS (800 micrograms)

Day 15: Follow-up; repeat ultrasound if abortion not confirmed at prior visit:
- If gestational cardiac activity present, perform D&C
- If only sac present, return in 3 weeks (day 36); if sac still present, counsel regarding D&C OR returning every 2 weeks for repeat ultrasound

INSTRUCTIONS FOR PATIENT

- Expect moderate (occasionally severe) cramping, bleeding and nausea
- Call or seek help if heavy bleeding (soaking 4 sanitary pads within 2 hours)
- Abstain from sexual intercourse, alcohol, and vitamins or folate supplements during treatment
- Either return for MIS or take it at home as directed
- Use acetaminophen or NSAIDs for analgesia; use codeine if inadequate relief
- Have a support person close by after MIS is given

PROBLEM MANAGEMENT

Pain - Oral analgesics, including NSAIDs; 1/300 women needs parenteral analgesia *[Creinin, 1997]*
Bleeding - D&C only for hemorrhage, or anemia requiring transfusion
Nausea/vomiting/diarrhea - Rarely requires treatment; if needed, use antiemetics & Lomotil

FERTILITY AFTER USE

- Immediate return to baseline fertility. Contraceptive should be supplied immediately
- No evidence of harm in future pregnancies due to these medications

EARLY MEDICAL ABORTION WITH MISOPROSTOL ALONE

Misoprostol is a prostaglandin analogue which causes very strong uterine contractions and can terminate pregnancy after 2-3 doses of 400-800 micrograms each

- Studies with misoprostol alone show efficacy of 68-94% up to 49 days, only 47-88% up to 56 days
- Given the inconsistancy of complete abortion rates when vaginal misoprostol is used alone, as well as the existence of safe alternative regimens, it generally is not recommended for medical abortions in the first trimester *[Goldberg, Greenberg and Darney - NEJM Jan 2001]*

Couples considering contraceptives and their health care providers face myriad questions about the *timing* of contraceptive use. Sometimes our clients come to us with mistaken ideas. *Sometimes we providers are actually the source of the misinformation.* In either case, timing errors, misconceptions, rigidity and oversimplifications can cause trouble. And *trouble* in family planning often can be spelled *unintended pregnancy*. Often it is overly dogmatic timing advice that causes trouble. In most instances, more important than advice about the *timing* of contraceptives is rapid initiation and then correct, *consistent use* of contraceptives. Below are several suggestions to consider in helping patients with timing questions:

1. For many women, a practical way to **start pills or the patch is on the first day of the next period**. Even easier, sometimes, is the Quick Start method which is to start pills on the day you first see a patient if you can be reasonably certain that she is not pregnant *[Westhoff 2002].* Recommend backup method for 7 days unless pills started on first day ◄— of menses or within 5 days of miscarriage

2. Healthy women who do not smoke can **continue pills indefinitely or until menopause** ◄— as long as they are not experiencing side effects or complications or develop contraindications. Encouraging women to take periodic "breaks" from taking pills, still recommended by some clinicians, is an unwise practice that can lead to unintended pregnancies

3. **Continuous use of combined pills with no pill free interval** is an acceptable way for some women to take pills

4. **The first Depo-Provera injection may be given at any time in the cycle** if a woman is not pregnant. If the day of the first shot is NOT within 5 days of the start of a period, recommend that patient use a back-up contraceptive for 7 days; some clinicians would ◄— recommend a repeat pregnancy test in 2-3 weeks

5. **Avoid overly dogmatic advice regarding when postpartum women should start progestin-only pills and the progestin-only injection, Depo-Provera.** There are clinicians and entire programs starting these two methods in each of the following 3 ways:
   • At discharge from hospital
   • 3 weeks postpartum
   • 6 weeks postpartum, but only if breastfeeding

6. **Recommend that condoms be placed onto the erect penis *OR* onto the penis *before* it becomes erect.** There are clear advantages and disadvantages to both approaches. Include both options in your written and oral instructions for patients

7. **Offer Plan B (emergency contraceptive pills) to women in advance.** Advance prescription of Plan B or Preven is one approach. Better yet, hand her the actual pills and instructions

8. **Copper intrauterine contraceptives may be inserted at any time in a woman's menstrual cycle** if she is not pregnant. Backup recommended for 7 days if not inserted in first 7 days

9. If in doubt about any timing question, **use condoms until your timing questions have been resolved**

CHAPTER 13

Choosing Among Available Methods
www.managingcontraception.com/choices
www.plannedparenthood.org/library

THE BEST METHOD IS THE ONE THAT IS MEDICALLY APPROPRIATE AND IS USED EVERY TIME BY SOMEONE HAPPY WITH THE METHOD

- Be aware of your own biases
- Each contraceptive method has both advantages and disadvantages
- Effectiveness and safety are important (see Tables 13.2, p. 38 and 13.3, p. 39)
- Convenience and ability to use method may determine effectiveness
- Protection against STIs/HIV needs to be considered for women and men at risk
- Effects of method on menses may be very important to a woman
- Ability to negotiate with partner may help determine method and selection
- Other influences (religion, privacy, past experience, friend's advice, frequency of intercourse) impact patient's preferences
- Discuss all methods with patient, even those you may not use in your own practice
- Consider discussing with couple, particularly if there appears to be conflict
- Ask if partner is supportive of contraception and condoms and whether he will pay for ← her contraception. Discuss cost of method and how she will pay for it ←

EFFECTIVENESS: measured by failure rates in 2 ways (see Table 13.2, p. 38)
Correct and consistent use first year failure rate: The percentage of women who become pregnant during their first year of use when they use the method correctly and consistently.
Typical use first year failure rates: The percentage of women who become pregnant during their first year of use. This number reflects the percent both of couples who use the method correctly and consistently and of those who do not. **This typical use failure rate is the relevant number to use when counseling new start users.**

- Failure rates may include previous users, restarters, or new users
- In spite of many very effective options, the U.S. has a high rate of unintended pregnancy. Approximately 50% of all pregnancies in the U.S. are not planned. Our challenge is to ← help women and couples use more effectively already available methods

KEY QUESTIONS
- *What contraceptive did you come to this office today wanting to use?*
- *Do you plan to have children? OR Do you plan to have more children?*
  If she says she wants no further pregnancies, be sure to discuss sterilization in addition to the highly effective reversible methods.
- *When (if ever) do you want to have your next child?*
  Helps teach need for preconceptional care and guides in selection of method
- *Does your partner want to have children in the future? When?*
- *What would you do if you had an accidental pregnancy? Is abortion an option?*

- *What are you doing to protect yourself from STIs/AIDS?*

  Inclusion of counseling about safer sex practices and condoms may be critical

- *Would you like to learn about emergency contraception?*

  Would she like a package of ECPs or a prescription for ECPs?

- *Do you have any serious medical problems?*

TABLE 13.1 Comparative risk of unprotected intercourse on unintended pregnancies and STI infections*

Unintended pregnancy/coital act	PID per woman infected with cervical gonorrhea
17%-30% midcycle	40% if not treated
<1% during menses	0% if promptly and adequately treated

Gonococcal transmission/coital act	Tubal infertility per PID episode
50% infected male, uninfected female	8% after first episode
25% infected female, uninfected male	20% after second episode
	40% after three or more episodes

Cates W Jr. Reproductive tract infections. In: Hatcher RA, et al. Contraceptive Technology. 17th ed. New York: Ardent Media, 1998:181.

Should Accutane (isotretinoin) be withheld from young reproductive-age women? No, but should be used very cautiously ◀

Accutane (isotretinoin) is a vitamin A isomer used in the treatment of extremely severe acne. It should only be used if a woman's acne is severe. If taken by a woman who is pregnant, it may cause a wide range of teratogenic effects from:

CNS: hydrocephalus, facial nerve palsy, cortical blindness and retinal defects AND

Craniofacial: low-set ears, microcephaly, triangular skull and cleft palate to

Cardiovascular: transposition of the great vessels, atrial and ventricular septal defects

Important contraceptive messages for women considering Accutane use, in view of the fact that no method of birth control is 100% effective

- **Use Two Methods:** In addition to compulsively careful and consistent use of a very effective hormonal contraceptive or intrauterine device, also use condoms consistently and correctly

- **Repeated Pregnancy Tests:** Pregnancy tests are essential prior to initiating and on a monthly basis thereafter. This is particularly important since the critical time of exposure to Accutane is believed to be 2-5 weeks after conception *[Briggs-2002]*

- **Consider Abortion if Contraceptive Failure:** Should pregnancy occur, strongly consider having an abortion performed. It is clear that this is happening. In the 22 months following its introduction, the manufacturer, FDA and CDC received reports on 154 Accutane-exposed pregnancies, of which 95 (61.7%) were electively aborted. Another 12 (7.8%) aborted spontaneously. 26 were born without major defects and 21 had major malformations *[Briggs-2002]*

- **Use Accutane Sparingly:** This drug is so dangerous to a developing fetus that it should not be used unless it is really necessary for disfiguring acne AND unless the reproductive-age women using it agrees to use two contraceptives consistently and correctly.

  Some clinicians would not provide this drug unless the woman using it agreed to have an abortion should a pregnancy exposed to Accutane occur

Table 13.2 Percentage of women experiencing an unintended pregnancy within the first year of typical use and the first year of perfect use and the percentage continuing use at the end of the first year: United States*

Method	% of Women Experiencing an Unintended Pregnancy within the First Year of Use		% of Women Continuing Use at One Year[1]
	Typical Use[2]	Perfect Use[3]	
No Method[4]	85	85	
Spermicides[5]	29	15	42
Withdrawal	27	4	43
Periodic Abstinence			51
Calendar	25	9	
Ovulation Method	25	3	
Symptothermal[6]	25	2	
Post-ovulation	25	1	
Cervical Cap with spermicide			
Parous Women	32	26	46
Nulliparous Women	16	9	57
Diaphragm with spermicide[7]	16	6	57
Condom[8]			
Reality Female Polyurethane condom	21	5	49
Male (Latex or polyurethane)	15	2	53
Pill	8	0.3	68
Ortho Evra patch	Unknown	0.3	68
NuvaRing	Unknown	0.3	68
Depo-Provera injections - q.3 months	3	0.3	56
Lunelle monthly injection	3	0.05	56
IUD			
Copper T (Paragard)	0.8	0.6	78
Levonorgestrel-releasing (Mirena)	0.1	0.1	81
Female Sterilization	0.5	0.5	100
Male Sterilization	0.15	0.10	100

Emergency Contraceptive Pills: Treatment with COCs initiated within 120 hours after unprotected intercourse reduces the risk of pregnancy by at least 60-75%.[9] Pregnancy rates lower if initiated in first 12 hours. Progestin-only EC reduces pregnancy risk by 89%.

Lactational Amenorrhea Method: LAM is a highly effective, temporary method of contraception.[10]

1 Among couples attempting to avoid pregnancy, the percentage who continue to use a method for 1 year

2 Among typical couples who initiate use of a method (not necessarily for the first time), the percentage who experience an accidental pregnancy during the first year if they do not stop use for any other reason

3 Among couples who initiate use of a method (not necessarily for the first time) and who use it perfectly (both consistently and correctly), the percentage who experience an accidental pregnancy during the first year if they do not stop use for any other reason

4 The percentages becoming pregnant in columns 2 and 3 are based on data from populations where contraception is not used and from women who cease using contraception in order to become pregnant. Among such populations, about 89% become pregnant within 1 year. This estimate was lowered slightly (to 85) to represent the percentages who would become pregnant within 1 year among women now relying on reversible methods of contraception if they abandoned contraception altogether

5 Foams, creams, gels, vaginal suppositories, and vaginal film

6 Cervical mucus (ovulation) method supplemented by calendar in the pre-ovulatory and basal body temperature in the post-ovulatory phases

7 With spermicidal cream or jelly

8 With or without spermicides (No difference in efficacy)

9 The treatment schedule is one dose within 72 hours after unprotected intercourse, and a second dose 12 hours after the first dose. See page 70 for pills that may be used

10 However, to maintain effective protection against pregnancy, another method of contraception must be used as soon as menstruation resumes, the frequency or duration of breast-feedings is reduced, bottle feeds are introduced, or the baby reaches 6 months of age

*Adapted from Trussell J, Kowal D. The essentials of contraception. In: Hatcher RA, et al. *Contraceptive Technology*, 18th ed. New York: Ardent Media, 2004.

Table 13.3 Major methods of contraception and some related safety concerns, side effects, and noncontraceptive benefits

[a]Trussell J, Kowal D. The essentials of contraception. IN: Hatcher RA, et al. *Contraceptive Technology*. 17th ed. New York: Ardent Media, 1998:235. Slight adaptations from CT table.

METHOD	COMPLICATIONS	SIDE EFFECTS	NONCONTRACEPTIVE BENEFITS *
Combined pills, injections, patch and ring	Cardiovascular complications (DVT, PE, MI, hypertension), depression, hepatic adenoma, slight increase in adenocarcinoma of cervix	Nausea, vomiting, headaches, dizziness, mastalgia, chloasma, spotting and bleeding, mood changes including, severe depression (rare)	Decreased dysmenorrhea, PMS, and blood loss; protects against symptomatic PID requiring hospitalization, ovarian and endometrial carcinomas, some benign tumors (leiomyomata, benign breast masses), ectopic pregnancies and ovarian cysts; reduces acne
Progestin-only pills	None	Spotting, breakthrough bleeding, amenorrhea, mood changes, headaches, hot flashes	Lactation not disturbed. Decreased menstrual pain & blood loss
Progestin-only implants	Infection at implant site, reaction to anesthesia, complicated removal, depression	Menstrual changes, mood changes, weight gain or loss, headaches, hair loss	Lactation not disturbed. Less blood loss per cycle. Reduced risk of ectopic pregnancy
Progestin-only injections	Allergic reaction, possible weight gain, glucose intolerance, depression	Menstrual changes, weight gain, headaches, hair loss, adverse impact on lipids, mood changes including, severe depression (rare)	Lactation not disturbed. Reduces risk of sickle cell crises, endometrial cancer, ovarian cysts, mittelschmerz. May reduce risk of PID, seizures, ovarian cancer. Can be used with anti-convulsants
IUD	PID following insertion, uterine perforation, bleeding with expulsion	Copper-IUD increases menstrual flow, blood loss and cramping; LNg IUD may cause irregular bleeding/amenorrhea	Lactation not disturbed. Copper T & levonorgestrel IUDs reduce risk for ectopic preg. Levonorgestrel IUD reduces cramping & pain & treats bleeding from DUB, menorrhagia, & fibroids
Sterilization	Surgical complications: hemorrhage, infection, organ damage, anesthetic complications, pain, ectopic pregnancy	Pain at surgical site, adhesion formation, subsequent regret	Women: reduced risk of ovarian cancer, endometrial cancer, ectopic pregnancy, PID Men: none known
Abstinence	None known	None except possible peer pressure; Partner may seek sex elsewhere	Prevents most STIs, cervical dysplasia; enhanced self-image possible
Male latex condom	Rare anaphylactic reactions to latex (use polyurethane)	Decrease in spontaneity; allergic reaction to latex, skin irritation	Reduces risk of STIs and cervical dysplasia
Female condom	TSS (although no cases reported)	Difficult to use, vaginal and bladder infection	May reduce STI and cervical dysplasia risk
Diaphragm Cervical cap	TSS, anaphylactic reaction to latex	Vaginal and bladder infection, vaginal erosions from poorly fit device, allergy to spermicide/latex. Diaphragms increase UTIs	Reduces risk of cervical STIs, PID and possibly cervical dysplasia

DESCRIPTION

Surveys reveal a wide variety of opinions about what constitutes sexual activity. However, from a family planning perspective, the definition of abstinence is clear: it is the absence of genital contact that could permit a pregnancy (i.e. penile penetration into the vagina). Some authors argue that abstinence is not a form of contraception, but is a lifestyle choice because an abstinent person is not having sex and, therefore, needs no contraception. Regardless, abstinence is an important means of reducing unintended pregnancies. A woman or a man may return to abstinence at any time. Abstinence-only-until-marriage education programs receive more than $100 million annually in government funds, most of it stemming from the Personal Responsibility and Work Opportunity Reconciliation Act of 1996. There is currently no evidence that any of these programs, which promote sexual abstinence and restrict information about contraception, actually achieve their intended purposes.

EFFECTIVENESS

Perfect use failure rate in first year: 0%
Typical use failure rates in first year: Unknown

MECHANISM

Sperm excluded from female reproductive tract, preventing fertilization

COST: None, except expense of pregnancy or pregnancy termination if plans change

ADVANTAGES: Can be restarted at any time! ←

Menstrual: none
Sexual/psychological:
• Can increase self esteem and positive self image if consistent with personal values
Cancers, tumors, and masses:
• Risk of cervical dysplasia far less if no vaginal intercourse has ever occurred
Other:
• Reduces risk of STIs (varies by what other sexual practices involved)
• Many religions and cultures endorse (at various stages in an individual's life)

DISADVANTAGES

Menstrual: None
Sexual/psychological:
• Frustration or sense of rejection if abstinence not self-selected
Cancers, tumors, and masses: None except indirectly. Virgins obviously remain nulliparous and, because of their nulliparity until an older age, have an increased risk for breast and ← ovarian cancer
Other:
• Requires commitment and self control; nonunderstanding partner may seek other partner(s)
• Patient and her partner may not be prepared to contracept if they stop abstaining

COMPLICATIONS

• No medical complications
• Person may be in situation where she/he wants to abstain, but partner does not agree. Women have been raped/beaten for refusing to have intercourse. Clearly, this is wrong. Occasionally there are dire consequences from the decision not to have intercourse.

CANDIDATES FOR USE

- Individuals or couples who feel they have ability to refrain from sexual intercourse

Adolescents:
- Very appropriate method but need to learn negotiating skills to effectively use abstinence and obtain information about contraceptive methods for future
- Counseling may include discussions on masturbation (solo or mutual) and also "outercourse" alternative ways of expressing affection/attraction/sexuality with partner

INITIATING METHOD

- Provide negotiating skills, how to say no, and how to resist peer (societal) pressures
- Recommend that patient ensure that partner explicitly agrees to abstain
- Can use abstinence at any time in life

INSTRUCTIONS FOR PATIENT

- Establish ground rules for herself and partner
- Prepare for time when (or if) decision to stop abstaining arises, initiate contraceptive counseling now
- Have condoms and emergency contraception on hand in case of need

PROBLEM MANAGEMENT

Partner does not want to abstain:
- Consider counseling in negotiating skills, role playing exercises and couple's counseling ◄
- Provide counseling in other forms of sexual pleasuring if patient interested (masturbation or outercourse)
- Seriously consider another birth control method or another partner!

FERTILITY AFTER USE

- Protects against upper reproductive tract infection preserving a woman's fertility
- Patient's baseline fertility (ability to cause pregnancy or become pregnant) is not altered if patient decides to have intercourse

---

Are Abstinence-Only Education Programs Effective?

According to a recent literature review conducted by Kirby (2001) for the National Campaign to Prevent Teen Pregnancy, only three evaluation studies of abstinence-only programs met the criteria established for inclusion in the review (e.g. random assignment, large sample size, long-term follow-up, measurement of behavior). All three studies measured program impact on the initiation of sex or frequency of sex. **None of the studies demonstrated a significant programmatic effect on the initiation of sex, frequency of sexual activity, or the number of sexual partners.** Although the results are not encouraging based on these three studies, Kirby concludes that there is insufficient evidence that abstinence-only programs do or do not delay sexual behavior. Large-scale evaluation data of the federally funded abstinence-only programs that resulted from the 1996 welfare reform act are expected at the end of 2002.

Source: Kirby, D. (2001). Emerging Answers: Research Findings on Programs to Reduce Teen Pregnancy. Washington, DC: The National Campaign to Prevent Teen Pregnancy.

CHAPTER 15

DESCRIPTION

In general, breastfeeding delays the return of fertility postpartum. However, LAM is a contraceptive method based on exclusively breast-feeding. LAM is an effective method only under specific conditions:

- Woman breast-feeding exclusively; both day and night feedings (at least 90% of baby's nutrition derived from breast-feeding)
- The woman is amenorrheic (spotting which occurs in the first 56 days postpartum is not regarded as menses)
- The infant is less than 6 months old

In the U.S., the median duration of breast-feeding is about 3 months. It is wise to provide a woman with another method to use when she no longer fulfills all the conditions. The probability that ovulation will precede the first menstrual period in a lactating woman increases from 33-45% during the first 3 months to 64-71% during months 4 to 12 and 87% after 12 months. *[Kennedy K.I. IN Hatcher RA Contraceptive Technology 17th Edition]*. Among lactating women, 66% are sexually active in the first month postpartum and 88% are sexually active in the second month postpartum *[Ford - 1998]*.

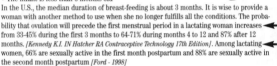

EFFECTIVENESS *[Kennedy - 1998]*

Perfect use failure rate in first 6 months: 0.5%
Typical use failure rate in first 6 months: 2%
At any time a woman is concerned, emergency contraception may be used by a nursing mother (preferably with levonorgestrel-only pills)

MECHANISM: Baby suckling on the mother's nipples causes a surge in maternal prolactin, which inhibits estrogen production and ovulation

COST: None

ADVANTAGES

NOTE: Most advantages and disadvantages are attributable to breastfeeding itself. The additional benefits accruing to LAM as a contraceptive method are minimal except convenience
Menstrual: Involution of the uterus occurs more rapidly; suppresses menses
Sexual/psychological: Breast-feeding pleasurable to many women

- Facilitates bonding between mother and child (if not stressful)

Cancers, tumors, and masses: Reduces risk of ovarian cancer and endometrial cancer; possible slight protective effect against breast cancer
Other:

- Can be used immediately after childbirth
- Provides the healthiest most "natural" food for baby
- Protects baby against asthma, allergies, URIs and diarrhea by passage of mother's antibodies into breastmilk
- Facilitates postpartum weight loss
- Less expensive and less time preparing bottles and feedings

DISADVANTAGES

Menstrual: Return to menses unpredictable
Sexual/psychological:

- Breastfeeding mother may be self-conscious in public or during intercourse
- Hypoestrogenism of breastfeeding may cause dyspareunia due to lack of lubrication

- Tender breasts may decrease sexual pleasure
- Women breastfeeding exclusively need lots of support from their partners in the home ◄

Cancers, tumors, and masses: None

Other:

- Working women need to find time/place/resources to pump ◄
- Effectiveness after 6 months is markedly reduced; return to fertility often precedes menses
- Frequent breastfeeding may be inconvenient or perceived as inconvenient
- No protection against STIs, HIV, AIDS
- If the mother is HIV+, there is a 14%-29% chance that HIV will be passed to infant via breast milk. Antiretroviral therapy decreases risk of transmission. Breastfeeding is ◄ not recommended for HIV+ women in the U.S.
- Sore nipples and breasts; risk of mastitis associated with breast-feeding

COMPLICATIONS: Mastitis risk increases and fertility can precede menses

CANDIDATES FOR USE

- Amenorrheic women less than 6 months postpartum who breast-feed their babies exclusively
- Women free of a blood borne infection which could be passed to the newborn
- Women not on drugs which can adversely affect their babies
- Adolescents may find this method difficult

MEDICAL ELIGIBILITY CHECKLIST

Ask the patient the questions below. If she answers "NO" to ALL questions, she can use LAM. If she answers Yes to any questions, follow the instructions. Sometimes there is a way to incorporate LAM into her contraceptive plans; in other situations, LAM is contraindicated.

1. Is your baby 6 months old or older?

☐ No ☐ Yes Help her choose another method to supplement the contraceptive effect of LAM

2. Has your menstrual period returned? (Bleeding in the first 8 weeks after childbirth does not count)

☐ No ☐ Yes After 8 weeks postpartum, if a woman has 2 straight days of menstrual bleeding, or her menstrual period has returned, she can no longer count on LAM as her contraceptive. Help her choose another method

3. Have you begun to breastfeed less often? Do you regularly give the baby other food or liquid (other than water)?

☐ No ☐ Yes If the baby's feeding pattern has just changed, explain that patient must be fully or nearly fully breastfeeding around the clock to protect against pregnancy. If not, she cannot use LAM effectively. Help her choose another method

4. Has a health-care provider told you not to breastfeed your baby?

☐ No ☐ Yes If a patient is not breastfeeding, she cannot use LAM. Help her choose another method. A woman should not breastfeed if she is taking mood altering recreational drugs, reserpine, ergotamine, antimetabolites, cyclosporine, bromocriptine, tetracycline, radioactive drugs, lithium, or certain anticoagulants (heparin and coumadin are safe); if her baby has a specific infant metabolic disorder; or possibly if she carries viral hepatitis or is HIV positive. All others can and should consider breastfeeding for the health benefits to the infant. In 1997, the FDA advised the manufacturer of Prozac (fluoxetine) to revise its labeling; it now states that "nursing while on Prozac is not recommended." On the other hand, Briggs notes that "the authors of a 1996 review stated that they encouraged women to continue breastfeeding while taking the drug" *[Nulman Tetralogy, 1996][Briggs, 2002]* This was also the conclusion of a 1999 review of the benefits of SSRIs for depressed breastfeeding women *[Edwards, 1999]*

5. Are you infected with HIV, the virus that causes AIDS?

☐ No ☐ Yes Where other infectious diseases kill many babies, mothers should be encouraged to breastfeed. HIV, however, may be passed to the baby in breast milk. When infectious diseases are a low risk and there is safe, affordable food for the baby, advise her to feed her baby that other food. Help her choose a birth control method other than LAM. A meta-analysis of published prospective trials estimated the risk of transmission of HIV with breastfeeding is 14% if the mother was infected prenatally but is 29% if the woman has her primary infection in the postpartum period

6. Do you know how long you plan to breastfeed your baby before you start supplementing his/her diet?

☐ No ☐ Yes In the U.S. the median duration of breastfeeding is approximately 3 months. Often breastfeeding women do not know when their menses will return, when they will start supplementing breastfeeding with other foods or exactly when they will stop breastfeeding their infant. It is wise to provide a woman with the contraceptive she will use when the answer to one of the above questions becomes positive and with a backup contraceptive and ECPs even during the period when she is breast-feeding is effective

INITIATING METHOD
- Patient should start exclusively breastfeeding immediately or as soon as possible after delivery
- Ensure that woman is breastfeeding fully or almost fully (>90% of baby's feedings); feedings around the clock
- Encourage use of second method of contraception if any questions about LAM effectiveness

INSTRUCTIONS FOR PATIENT
- Breastfeed consistently, exclusively and correctly for maximum effectiveness
- Breast milk should constitute at least 90% of baby's feedings
- Think about methods that can be used once menses return ◀

PROBLEM MANAGEMENT
Deficient milk supply:
- The more a breast is emptied, the more it fills up ◀
- Commonly caused by insufficient nursing, use of artificial nipple, fatigue or maternal stress
- Encourage woman to breastfeed often (8-10 times daily), eat well, get additional rest, drink lots of fluids and take prenatal vitamins and iron supplements
- Immediately postpartum women should breastfeed every 2-3 hours to stimulate milk production
- Avoid estrogen-containing contraceptives

Sore nipples:
- Provide good support of breasts and psyche (inform her about La Leche League and of other lactation specialists)
- Commonly caused by incorrect positioning of the baby to the breast. Uncommonly caused by infection
- Check for correct ways of latching and suckling; be sure to break the suction before removing the baby from the breast
- Improve with practice; change the pressure points on the nipple by changing the ◀ baby's position for feeding
- Allow nipples to air dry with breast milk on the areola to reduce infection and nipple soreness
- Do not cleanse breasts other than with water at any time
- Apply lanolin to nipples after each feeding to decrease soreness

Sore breasts:

- Wear a well-fitted, supportive nursing bra; avoid bras that are too tight or have underwire ◀
- Apply heat on sore areas; some women apply teabag as compress on sore nipples
- Nurse frequently or use pump to get excess milk out of affected breast
- Encourage additional rest
- Seek medical evaluation if any erythema, fever or other signs or symptoms of infection develop

Other:

- Stress, fear, lack of confidence, lack of strong motivation to succeed at breastfeeding, lack of partner and/or societal support, and/or poor nutrition can cause problems

FERTILITY AFTER USE

Patient's baseline fertility (ability to become pregnant) is not altered once patient discontinues breastfeeding

---

TEN STEPS TO SUCCESSFUL BREASTFEEDING

From: Protecting, Promoting and Supporting Breastfeeding: The special role of maternity services. (A joint WHO/UNICEF statement. Geneva, World Health Organization, 1989)

All healthcare facilities where childbirth is undertaken should:

1. Have a written breastfeeding policy that is routinely communicated to all health care staff.
2. Train all health care staff in skills necessary to implement this policy.
3. Inform all pregnant women about the benefits and management of breastfeeding.
4. Help mothers initiate breastfeeding within the first 30 minutes after birth.
5. Show mothers how to breastfeed and how to maintain lactation even if they are separated from their infants because of a medical reason.
6. Give newborn infants no milk feeds or water other than breast milk unless indicated for a medical reason.
7. Allow mothers and infants to remain together 24 hours a day from birth.
8. Encourage natural breastfeeding on demand.
9. Do not give or encourage the use of artificial teats or dummies to breastfeed infants.
10. Promote the establishment of breastfeeding support groups and refer mothers to these on discharge from the hospital or clinic.

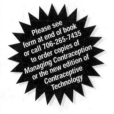

Please see form at end of book or call 706-265-7435 to order copies of Managing Contraception or the new edition of Contraceptive Technology

All breastfeeding women should be provided contraception because:
- Duration of breastfeeding in the U.S. is typically brief
- Most couples resume intercourse a few weeks after delivery
- Spacing of pregnancies is important to maternal and child health
- Ovulation may precede first menses

Table 16.1 *When to initiate contraception in breastfeeding women:*

METHOD	WHEN TO START IN LACTATING WOMEN	EFFECT ON BREAST MILK
Condoms (Male & Female), Sponge	• Immediately after lochia stops (intercourse prior to that time carries risk of infection)	No effect
Cervical Cap, Diaphragm	• 4-6 weeks postpartum, after cervix and vagina normalized (need to be refitted for postpartum women)	No effect
Progestin-Only Methods • Depo-Provera • Progestin - Only Pills • Norplant • Implanon	• Most authorities, including National Medical Committee of the Planned Parenthood Federation of America, consider it appropriate to initiate any progestin-only method immediately postpartum • WHO and International Planned Parenthood Federation recommend waiting 6 weeks postpartum because of theoretical concerns for the newborn infant	• No significant impact on milk quality or production • Breast-feeding prolonged • Breast fed children of DPMA users grow at normal rate • Lactation Specialists recommend that women starting DMPA/POPs should be informed that milk production may decrease in some women
Combined Pills or Combined Injections Patch Vaginal Ring	• American Academy of Pediatrics recommends use when infant's diet supplemented but no sooner than 3-6 weeks postpartum • Most conservative position: await weaning to avoid possible decrease in breast milk • Also, see Table 26.2 on pg. 105	Quality and quantity of breast milk may be diminished if used prior to establishment of lactation. After lactation establishment, COCs have no significant impact
IUD: • Copper • Levonorgestrel	• Usually await uterine involution to insert (4-6 weeks) • May insert Copper or LNg IUD within first 20 minutes after delivery of placenta with special equipment	No effect with Copper IUD; theoretical effect as above for Mirena
Tubal Sterilization	Usually done in first 24-48 hours postpartum, or await complete uterine involution for interval tubal sterilization (> 6 weeks postpartum)	No effect

Fertility Awareness Methods (FAM) & Periodic Abstinence

www.dml.georgetown.edu/depts/irh OR www.usc.edu/hsc/info/newman/resource/nfp.html
www.cyclebeads.com OR www.irh.org OR info@cyclebeads.com

DESCRIPTION: A woman cannot identify the exact day of ovulation using FAM methods; rather she identifies when the fertile phase of her cycle begins and ends. A woman's fertile phase may begin 3-5 days before ovulation (because sperm can live in cervical mucus for 3-5 days); a woman's fertile phase ends 24 hours after ovulation

For purposes of FAM, a woman's menstrual cycle has 3 phases:
1. Infertile phase: before ovulation
2. Fertile phase: Approximately 5-7 days in the mid-portion of the cycle, including several days before and the day of ovulation;
3. Infertile phase: after ovulation

Of the FAM methods discussed, the Calendar Method, Standard Days Method, and the Cervical Mucus Method can be used to identify the beginning and the end of the fertile period; the BBT Method can only be used to identify the end of the fertile period. Thus, couples using the BBT Method could only safely have unprotected intercourse during the post-ovulatory period, as the method cannot be used to define the pre-ovulatory infertile phase. As couples using either the Calendar or the Cervical Mucus Methods can theoretically identify the beginning and the end of the fertile period, they may have unprotected intercourse during the pre-ovulatory infertile phase and the post-ovulatory infertile phase. However, in order to minimize the chance of an unintended pregnancy, some advocate that couples only have unprotected intercourse during the post-ovulatory infertile phase regardless of the method of FAM they are using.

Techniques used to determine high-risk fertile days include:

1. Calendar Method
- Record days of menses prospectively for 6 cycles
- Most estimates assume that sperm can survive 2-3 days and ovulation occurs 14 days before menses (motile sperm have been found as long as 7 days after intercourse and the extreme interval following a single act of coitus leading to an achieved pregnancy is 6 days [Speroff-1999])
- Earliest day of fertile period = day # in a cycle corresponding to **shortest cycle length minus 18**
- Latest day of fertile period = day # in a cycle corresponding to **longest cycle length minus 11**

2. Standard Days Method
- For women with cycles 26-32 days long, avoid intercourse on days 8-19 (white beads on CycleBead necklace). No need for 3-6 months of extensive cycle calculations
- 4.75% failure over 1 year with perfect use; 11.96% with typical use [Arevalo-2002]
- Resources available from the Institute for Reproductive Health, www.irh.org (CD, training manual, patient brochure, sample beads). Beads can also be ordered from www.cyclebeads.com

3. Cervical Mucus Ovulation Detection Method
- Women check quantity and character of mucus on the vulva or introitus with fingers or tissue paper each day for several months to learn cycle:

  - Post-menstrual mucus: scant or undetectable
  - Pre-ovulation mucus: cloudy, yellow or white, sticky
  - Ovulation mucus: clear, wet stretches, sticky (but slippery)
  - Post-ovulation fertile mucus: thick, cloudy; less
  - Post-ovulation post-fertile mucus: scant or undetectable
- When using method during preovulatory period, must abstain 24 hours after intercourse to make test interpretable as semen and vaginal fluids can obscure character of cervical mucus
- Abstinence or barrier method through fertile period (ie abstinence for a given cycle begins as soon as the woman notices any cervical secretions)
- Intercourse without restriction beginning 4th day after the last day of wet, clear, slippery mucus

4. Basal Body Temperature Method (BBT)

- Assumes early morning temperature measured before arising will increase noticeably (0.4-0.8° F) with ovulation; fertile period is defined as the day of first temperature drop or first elevation through 3 consecutive days of elevated temperature. Temperature drop does NOT always occur

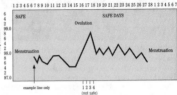

Days of Menstrual Cycle

Figure 17.1 Basal body temperature variations during a menstrual cycle

- Abstinence begins first day of mentrual bleeding and lasts through 3 consecutive days of sustained temperature rise

5. Post-ovulation Method

- Permits unprotected intercourse only after signs of ovulation have subsided

6. Symptothermal Method

- Combines at least two methods — usually cervical mucus changes with BBT
- May also include mittelschmerz, change in libido, and changes in cervical texture, position and dilation to detect ovulation:
  - During preovulatory and ovulatory periods, cervix softens, opens and is moister
  - During postovulatory period, cervix drops, becomes firm and closes

EFFECTIVENESS (see Table 13.2, page 36)

NFP/FAM First-year failure rate (100 women-years of use)

Method	Typical use*	Perfect use
Calendar	25	9
Ovulation Method	25	3
Symptothermal	25	2
Post-ovulation	25	1

*FAM usually more effective than NFP   *[Trussell IN Contraceptive Technology, 2003]*

MECHANISM: Abstinence or barriers during fertile period

COST: Training, supplies (special digital basal body thermometer), and barriers

ADVANTAGES

Menstrual:

- No change
- Helps woman learn more about her menstrual physiology

Sexual/psychological: Men and women can work together in using this method. Men must be aware that abstinence or use of second method is essential during the fertile period

Cancers, tumors, and masses: None

Other:

- May be only method acceptable to couples for cultural or religious reasons
- Helps couples achieve pregnancy when practiced in reverse

DISADVANTAGES

Menstrual:

- Difficult to use in early adolescence, when approaching menopause, and in postpartum women when cycles are irregular (or absent), or with vaginal infections
- Even women with "regular" periods can vary as much as ± 7 days in any given cycle

Sexual/psychological:
- Requires abstinence, barrier method, or another contraceptive that does not change pattern of ovulation during 6-12 month learning/data-gathering period unless CycleBead method is used ◄—
- Complete abstinence in an ovulatory cycle, if using post-ovulation techniques. This ◄— method demands great self-control: either abstinence or use of another method must be used during long periods of time when woman is or may be fertile
- Requires discipline, good communication and full commitment of both partners
- Requires abstinence at time of ovulation, which is the time of peak libido

Cancers, tumors, and masses: None

Other:
- May not be helpful during time of stress
- Method very unforgiving of improper use
- Does not protect against STIs
- Relatively high failure rate with typical use
- Less reliable in settings of fever, vaginal infections, douching, spermicides, and certain medications

COMPLICATIONS: None

CANDIDATES FOR USE
- Women with regular, predictable menstrual cycles
- Those with religious/cultural proscriptions against using other methods
- Those meeting medical eligibility criteria
- Highly motivated couples willing to commit to extensive abstinence or to use barriers during vulnerable periods

Adolescents: Not appropriate until regular menstrual cycles established

MEDICAL ELIGIBILITY CHECKLIST
Ask the woman the questions below. If she answers NO to ALL questions, she CAN use any fertility awareness-based method if she wants. If she answers YES to any question, follow the instructions. No conditions restrict use of these methods, but some conditions can make them harder to use effectively

1. Do you have a medical condition that would make pregnancy especially dangerous?

    ☐ No   ☐ Yes   She may want to choose a more effective method. If not, stress careful use of fertility awareness-based methods to avoid pregnancy and availability of EC

2. Do you have irregular or prolonged menstrual cycles? Vaginal bleeding between periods?
*   For younger women: Are your periods just starting?*
*   For older women: Have your periods become irregular?*

    ☐ No   ☐ Yes   Predicting her fertile time with only the calendar method may be hard or impossible. She can use basal body temperature (BBT) and/or cervical mucus, or she may prefer another method

3. Did you recently give birth or have an abortion? Are you breastfeeding?
*   Do you have any other condition that affects menstrual bleeding?*

    ☐ No   ☐ Yes   These conditions may affect fertility signs, making fertility awareness-based methods hard to use. For this reason, a woman or couple may prefer a different method. If not, they may need more counseling and follow-up to use the method effectively

☐ No ☐ Yes If her cycles have not been re-established, she may need to use another method until cycles are regular

☐ No ☐ Yes These conditions may affect fertility signs, making fertility awareness-based methods hard to use. Once an infection is treated and reinfection is avoided, however, a woman can use fertility awareness-based methods more easily

INITIATING METHOD

• Requires several months of data collection and analysis unless using CycleBeads ◄——
• Description of methods
• Formal training necessary. Couples may be trained together
• Resources are available from:
  1. Calgary Billings Centre of Natural Family Planning, Room 1, 1247 Bel-Aire Dr SW, Calgary, AB T2V 2C1, (403) 252-3929, www.billings-centre.ab.ca
  2. California Association of Natural Family Planning, 1010 - 11th St, Suite 200, Sacramento, CA 95814, (877) 332-2637, www.canfp.org
  3. The Couple to Couple League International, PO Box 111184, Cincinnati, OH 45211-1184, (513) 471-2000, www.ccli.org
  4. Institute for Reproductive Health, Georgetown University Medical Center, 3 PHC, Room 300r, 3800 Reservoir Rd, NW, Washington, DC 20007, (202) 687-1392, www.dml.georgetown.edu/depts/irh
  5. National Center for Women's Health, Pope Paul VI Institute, 6901 Mercy Road, Omaha, NE 68106-2604, (402) 390-6600, www.popepaulvi.com
  6. Family of the Americas Foundation, Inc., PO Box 1170, Dunkirk, MD 20754-1170, (800) 443-3395, www.familyplanning.net
  7. Northwest Family Services, 4805 NE Glisan St, Portland, OR 97213, (503) 230-6377, www.nwfs.org
  8. Twin Cities NFP Center, HealthEast, St. Joseph's Hospital, 69 W Exchange St, St. Paul, MN 55102, (651) 232-3088, www.tcnfp.org

INSTRUCTIONS FOR PATIENT

• Requires discipline, communication, listening skills, full commitment of both partners. Mistakes using this method are particularly likely to lead to unintended pregnancies ◄—— as intercourse is then occurring at the time in the cycle when a woman is *most* likely to become pregnant
• If using FAM, use contraception during fertile days
• If using NFP, abstain from sexual intercourse during fertile days
• Encourage other forms of sexual satisfaction

FOLLOW-UP

• Have you had sexual intercourse during "unsafe" times during your cycle?
• Discuss use of emergency contraception if having sex during "unsafe" times during cycle

PROBLEM MANAGEMENT

Inconsistent use and risk taking: Educate about emergency contraception when women start using method

FERTILITY AFTER USING: Return to baseline fertility

DESCRIPTION: Condoms for men are sheaths made of latex, polyurethane or natural membranes (usually lamb cecum), which are placed over the penis prior to genital contact and worn until after ejaculation when the penis is removed from the vagina or anus. Latex condoms are available in at least 2 sizes, in a wide variety of textures and thicknesses (0.03-0.09 mm), and come with or without spermicidal coating. Two brands of polyurethane condoms are currently available in the US. When used correctly and consistently, male latex condoms are effective in preventing sexual ◄ transmission of HIV and can reduce the risk for other STDs (ie gonorrhea, chlamydia and trichomonas). Natural membrane condoms may not provide that additional STI protection. Condoms may be used as a primary contraceptive method, as a back up method, or with another method to provide STI risk reduction. **When used as a primary contraceptive method, it is important that condoms be coupled with advance provision/prescription of emergency ◄ contraceptive pills (ECPs) since couples experience a condom break or slippage during approximately 3-5% of acts of intercourse:**

> If 14,000 acts of intercourse are protected by condoms, a mishap (breakage, slippage ◄ part of the way down the shaft of the penis, or slippage completely off the penis) will occur approximately 5% of the time or 700 times. If couples experiencing breakage or slippage identify this and use a single tablet of Plan B (0.75 mg levonorgestrel) within one hour, only one of those 700 women will experience an unintended pregnancy. The failure rate of a single tablet of Plan B within one hour of unprotected sex is 0.14% or just about 1 in 700 *[Shelton - 2002]*

EFFECTIVENESS *[Trussell J IN Contraceptive Technology, 2004]*
Perfect use failure rate in the first year of use: 2% (See Table 13.2, page 38)
Typical use failure rate in the first year of use: 15%
* The most common reason for condom failure is not using a condom ◄
* Comparative testing has shown that latex and polyurethane condoms provide the same pregnancy protection. However, there was a significant difference between the materials in slippage and breakage rates:

Condom Breakage and Slippage	Polyurethane	Latex
Trial 1	10.5%	1.7%
Trial 2	8.5%	1.6%

MECHANISM
* Condoms act as a mechanical barrier; they prevent the passage of sperm into the female reproductive tract. Sheathing the penis also reduces transmission and acquisition of STIs, including HIV. Spermicidal condoms are no longer recommended ◄

COST
* Average retail cost for latex condoms is $0.50, but some designer condoms cost several dollars. Polyurethane condoms cost $.80-$2.00 each
* Public health agencies often offer free condoms. Purchasers of large numbers of condoms may buy condoms for as low as 4 to 6 cents per condom from Ansell and Durex

ADVANTAGES
Menstrual: No direct impact on menses, but couple may feel more aesthetically comfortable
Sexual/psychological:
  * Some men may maintain erection longer with condoms, making sex more enjoyable
  * If the woman/partner puts the condom on, it may add to sexual pleasure
  * Male involvement is encouraged and is essential!
  * Availability of wide selection of condom types and designs can add variety

51

- Makes sex less messy by catching the ejaculate
- Intercourse may be more pleasurable because fear of pregnancy and STIs is decreased

Cancers/tumors & masses: Decrease in HIV transmission reduces risks of AIDS-related malignancies

Other:
- Significantly reduces risks of HIV transmission (Figure 18.2, p. 56) and some other STIs
- Readily available over the counter; no medical visit required
- Usually inexpensive for single use
- Easily transportable. Don't leave in wallet too long; probably ok for 1 month ←
- Opportunity for couples to improve communication and negotiating skills
- Immediately active after placement
- May reduce risk of PID, infertility, ectopic pregnancy and chronic pelvic pain

DISADVANTAGES

Menstrual: None

Sexual/psychological:
- Use may interrupt or be perceived as interrupting lovemaking. Requires discipline to resist impulse to progress to intercourse after erection
- May cause man to lose erection
- Blunting of sensation or "unnatural" feeling with intercourse
- Plain condoms may decrease lubrication and provide less stimulation for woman (use water-based or silicone lubricant with latex condoms if this is a problem)
- Requires prompt withdrawal after ejaculation, which may decrease pleasure
- Makes sex messier (getting rid of condom)

Cancers/tumors and masses: None

Other:
- Requires education/experience for successful use
- Either member of couple may have latex allergy or reaction to spermicide (polyurethane condom is appropriate alternative)
- Users must avoid petroleum-based vaginal products when using latex condoms (Figure 18.1, p. 55) (polyurethane condom is appropriate alternative)
- Couples may be embarrassed to purchase or to apply condoms due to taboos about touching genitalia, stigma of concern about STDs/HIV

COMPLICATIONS

- Allergic reactions to latex are rarely life threatening; 2-3% of Americans (men and women) have a latex allergy; up to 14% of latex workers are latex sensitive. Polyurethane condoms do not cause allergic reactions
- Condom retained in vagina (uncommon) exposes woman to risk of infection as well as pregnancy. If this occurs: 1) try to remove by pinching with second and third fingers or 2) enlist partner's help or 3) go to clinician ASAP. Use EC ASAP

PRECAUTIONS

- Men who are unable to maintain erection when they wear condoms; benzocaine ← condoms by Durex are now available. Benzocaine is to prevent premature ejaculation
- Men with abnormal ejaculatory pathways not sheathed by condom
- Woman whose partners will not use condoms
- Women who require high contraceptive efficacy should, at a minimum, add another method in addition to the condom
- Couples in which either partner has latex allergy should avoid latex condoms (men can use Durex-Avanti or Trojan-Supra; women can use Reality female condom)
- Couples in which either partner has spermicide allergy or is at high risk for HIV should avoid ← spermicide-coated condoms

CANDIDATES FOR USE

- Anyone at risk for an STI
- Appropriate for most couples
- May be used alone or coupled with a second contraceptive method

Special applications for infection control:
  - Non-monogamous couples (i.e. if either partner has multiple partners)
  - During pregnancy as well as at all other times
  - After delivery or loss to reduce risk of endometritis (although abstinence is better) ◄
  - Couples with known viral infections (HIV, HPV, HSV-2) in areas sheathed by device

Adolescents: Excellent option, especially when combined with another method

INITIATING METHOD

Couples desiring to use condoms often benefit from concrete instructions. Use a model and actual condom. Counsel new users about:
- Options among condom types
- Storage for safety and ready access
- How to negotiate condom use with partner and when to place condom
- How to open package and place correct side of condom over penis
- How to unroll and allow space for ejaculate (depending on condom design)

Provide ECPs to couples relying on the condom for birth control to insure immediate use in the event of condom mishap or problem. This will minimize risk of unintended pregnancy

INSTRUCTIONS FOR PATIENTS (See Figure 18.1, pg. 55)

- Learn how to use a condom long before you need it. Both women and men need to know how. Practice with models: fingers, bananas or man's penis
- Buy condoms in advance, carry with you; Keep extra condoms out of sunlight and heat
- Try new condoms to find favorite size, scent, and texture and to add variety
- Check date on condom carefully. It may be an expiration date OR a date of production. If it is an expiration date, do not use beyond expiration date. If it is a date of production, condom may be used for several years from the date of production (2 years for spermicidal condoms, 5 years for nonspermicidal latex condoms)
- Open package carefully, squeeze condom out, avoid tearing with fingernails, teeth, etc.
- Use appropriate water-based or silicon-based lubricant with latex condoms (see page 55). Never put lubricant inside the condom

Researchers at Univ. Texas Galveston found 3 vaginal lubricants that are safe, non-irritating (unlike Nonoxynol-9) and strongly inhibited HIV replication in vitro: Astroglide, Vagisil and ViAmor. *[AIDS Research and Human Retroviruses-2001].* But beware: N-9 also inhibited ◄ HIV replication in vitro and see what happened with N-9 in vivo. More data needed

- Place condom over penis before any genital contact. Either partner can put it on!
- Consider placing a second condom (larger size) over lubricated condom if history of previous breakage or if man has any evidence of STI
- If condom used for oral or rectal intercourse replace with a new condom prior to vaginal entry
- Vigorous sex can be fun but can break the condom. Consider using 2 condoms at once
- Immediately after ejaculation (before loss of erection) hold rim of condom against shaft of penis and remove condom-covered penis from vagina (or anus)
- Remove condom from the penis and inspect carefully for any breaks
- Dispose of condom. Do not reuse
- If a condom falls off, slips, tears or breaks, apply vaginal spermicidal foam immediately and start using ECPs as soon as possible. If you do not have ECPs, call 1-888-NOT-2-LATE or check www.not-2-late.com to find out how to get them. In some states, you can gt EC ◄ from a pharmacist without a prescription. If any risk for STIs, seek medical care

53

FOLLOW-UP

- Are you and your partner comfortable using condoms?
- Have you had any problems with using the condom? Breaking? Slipping off? Decreased sensation? Vaginal soreness with use? Skin irritation or redness during the day after using it?
- Have you had any post-coital "yeast infection" symptoms? (A woman may confuse an allergic reaction to the condom and/or spermicide with a candidal infection)
- Have you had intercourse—even once—without a condom?
- Did you have any problems with ECPs?
- Do you need more ECPs?
- Do you plan to have children? OR Do you plan to have more children? When?

PROBLEM MANAGEMENT

Allergic reaction:
- Beware that latex powder can induce anaphylaxis and that the severity of allergic reaction can precipitously increase with continued exposure. Sometimes a person who says he (or she) is allergic to condoms may mean condoms are a) difficult to put on or b) lead to loss of erection or c) the couple simply doesn't like condoms or d) is being irritated ◄— by a spermicide or e) an ongoing infection may be causing irritation
- Switch to polyurethane condoms (Durex-Avanti or Trojan-Supra male condoms or Reality female condom) or stop using spermicide (depending on the suspected allergen)
- Switch to another method, such as the female condom for STI risk reduction and a hormonal method for contraception

Condom breakage: (Figure 18.3, p. 56) (1-2% for latex condoms)
- Insure correct technique. Common problems: pre-placement manipulations (stretching, etc), use of inappropriate lubricant, and prolonged or extremely vigorous sex
- May need to recommend larger condom
- If couple using polyurethane, consider switching to latex condom
- May need to switch method
- Confirm that woman is using ECPs and has supply available at home

Condom slippage: (Figure 18.3, p. 56) (More common than condom breakage)
- Ensure correct technique. Common problems: condom not fully unrolled, lubricant placed incorrectly on inside of condom, and excessive delay in removing penis from vagina after ejaculation. Use of proper-sized condom is important ◄—
- Rule out erectile dysfunction. Condoms may not be appropriate if man loses erection with condom placement or use
- Confirm that woman is using ECPs and has supply available at home

Decreased sensation:
- Common causes: condom too small, too thick or too tightly applied; inadequate lubrication
- Suggest experimentation with different textured condoms or placing second (larger size) condom over lubricated inner condom. Thinner condoms now available (Durex) ◄—
- Integrate condom placement into lovemaking (suggest partner place condom to help arouse/excite man)

FERTILITY AFTER USE

- Immediate return to baseline fertility
- May protect fertility by reducing risk of STIs

Figure 18.1

HOW TO USE A LATEX CONDOM
(...Or rubber, sheath, prophylactic, safe, french letter, raincoat, glove, sock)

Talk/Think about condom use with partner. Make the FIRM commitment, in advance, to use condoms without exception with each/every sexual act (vaginal, oral or anal)

↓

Keep a supply of condoms handy...Store condoms in a cool, dry place away from sunlight and check the expiration date **before** use

↓

Use NEW condom before any sexual contact

↓

USE CONDOM CORRECTLY.
Before putting on the condom, check to see which way the condom unrolls.
(If uncircumcised, pull back foreskin before unrolling condom.)
Unroll condom all the way down to the base of the penis (down to hair).
NOTE: A condom can be put onto a penis that is not fully erect.
Smooth out air bubbles. Make sure condom fits (condoms come in various sizes)

↓

Add WATER-based lubricant to outside of condom if desired

↓

Condom must be used throughout sex

↓

Change condom if sex prolonged or if penis exposed to different orifice

↓

After sex: Hold rim of condom and carefully withdraw penis before loss of erection

↓

RELAX. Check for breakage; Dispose of condom. (If condom breaks, slips, falls off or is not used, use EC. If not already available, call 1-888-NOT-2-LATE for Emergency Contraception.)
Wash areas exposed to body fluids (penis, vulva, etc.) with soap and water

---

SAFE!
WATER BASED OR SILICONE LUBRICANTS SAFE FOR USE WITH CONDOMS

Astroglide
Water and saliva
Glycerin
All I-D Lubricants
Aloe-9
H-R Lubricating Jelly
K-Y Jelly
Prepair
Probe
AquaLube
ForPlay
Gynol II
Wet
Cornhuskers Lotion
Silicone Lubricant
deLube
Spermicide *

* Spermicidal condoms are no longer recommended although spermicides do not damage latex

---

UNSAFE FOR USE WITH LATEX CONDOMS*

Aldara cream
Baby oil or Cold creams
Edible oils (olive, peanut, corn, sunflower)
Head and body lotions
Massage oils
Mineral oil
Petroleum jelly
Rubbing alcohol
Shortening
Suntan oil and lotions
Whipped cream
Vegetable oil and cooking oils
Cindamycin 2% vaginal cream
Vaginal yeast infection medications in cream or suppository form
• Butoconazole cream
• Clotrimazole cream
• Clotrimazole vaginal tablet
• Miconazole vaginal suppository
• Terconazole ointment
• Terconazole cream or vaginal suppository

These lubricants/vaginal products can be used with polyurethane condoms

55

Figure 18.2 10 Studies demonstrating protective effect of latex condoms in heterosexual couples

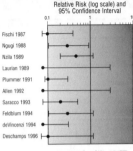

Relative Risk (log scale) and
95% Confidence Interval

Fischl 1987
Ngugi 1988
Nzila 1989
Laurian 1989
Plummer 1991
Allen 1992
Saracco 1993
Feldblum 1994
deVincenzi 1994
Deschamps 1996

[Feldblum et al., 1995]

Figure 18.3

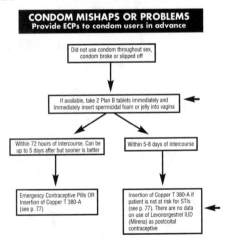

CONDOM MISHAPS OR PROBLEMS
Provide ECPs to condom users in advance

Did not use condom throughout sex, condom broke or slipped off

↓

If available, take 2 Plan B tablets immediately and Immediately insert spermicidal foam or jelly into vagina

Within 72 hours of intercourse. Can be up to 5 days after but sooner is better

Within 5-8 days of intercourse

Emergency Contraceptive Pills OR Insertion of Copper T 380-A (see p. 77)

Insertion of Copper T 380-A if patient is not at risk for STIs (see p. 77). There are no data on use of Levonorgestrel IUD (Mirena) as postcoital contraceptive

DESCRIPTION: The Reality Female-Intiated Condom

A condom inserted by women (or partner). Disposable, single-use polyurethane sheath, which is placed into the vagina. Flexible and movable inner ring at closed end is used to insert device into the vagina. Larger, fixed outer ring remains outside the vagina to cover part of introitus. Shelf life 3-5 years. When used as primary method, the female condom should be coupled with advance prescription of emergency contraceptive pills (ECPs)

EFFECTIVENESS [Trussell J. IN Contraceptive Technology, 2004]
Perfect use failure rate in first year of use: 5% (Table 13.2, pg. 38)
Typical use failure rate in first year of use: 21%

MECHANISM

- The female condom acts as a mechanical barrier; it prevents pregnancy by preventing the passage of sperm into the female reproductive tract
- Sheathing reduces transmission and acquisition of bacterial and viral STIs into the vagina and upper reproductive track

COST in 1995 [Trussell, 1995; Smith, 1993]

	Managed-Care Setting	Public Sector Setting
Published prices	$3.66	$1.25
Typical negotiated prices	$2.00-3.00	$0.70

ADVANTAGES

Menstrual: No impact on menses per se, but couple may feel more comfortable having intercourse during menses if a female condom is used

Sexual/psychology

- Intercourse may be more pleasurable because fear of pregnancy and STIs is decreased
- Can be inserted up to 8 hours before sex to allow more spontaneity
- If woman inserts it, she can be sure she is somewhat protected
- Makes sex less messy for the women after removal of the condom

Cancers/tumor, masses: no data

Other

- Available over-the-counter; no medical visit required
- Immediately active after placement
- Provides option to women whose partners can not or will not use male condom. May circumvent erectile concerns some men have with male condoms
- Although studies are lacking, is expected to reduce risk of fluid borne STI and HIV transmission and acquisition
- Can be safely used by people with latex allergies or sensitivities
- May possibly reuse for contraceptive purposes but NOT if being used to prevent infections. Reuse is generally not recommended. If women want to wash and reuse Reality condom, WHO recommendations are as follows:
  1) soak in bleach for 1 minute (kills HIV, HSV-2, CT, GC - 1 part bleach to 20 parts water) 2) Rinse with water 3) Wash gently with soap and water and pat dry 4) Store in clean, dry place. May reuse up to 5 times

DISADVANTAGES

Menstrual: None

Sexual/psychology:
- Use may interrupt lovemaking unless woman inserts beforehand in anticipation of intercourse
- Requires careful sexual practices during intercourse (see INSTRUCTIONS FOR PATIENT), which may make intercourse awkward and less spontaneous
- May be difficult for woman to ask her partner to follow instructions for use
- Noise made during intercourse may be distracting (additional lubricant can quiet)
➤ In one study, 88% of women disliked using the Reality Female Condom *[Duerr-Macaluso, 1999]*

Cancers/tumors/masses: None

Other:
- Somewhat difficult for new users (even experienced diaphragm users) to insert especially if woman is immediately postpartum ◄
- Requires application with each act of intercourse
- Requires education and experience for successful use
- Couples may be embarrassed to purchase and to apply condoms due to taboos about touching genitalia; stigma of concern about STDs/HIV
➤ Prostate Specific Antigen (PSA) found in the vagina of women following intercourse using the female condom indicates exposure to semen. PSA was found in the vagina after 7% of acts of SI and was more likely to occur in couples where the women's vaginal fundus was large, the man's penis was small, there was a high level of activity at the time of intercourse or partners had been in their current relationship for less than 2 years *[Lawson 2003]*

COMPLICATIONS: Intravaginal methods can change vaginal flora and increase UTI risks

PRECAUTIONS
- Women unable to insert condom correctly and follow other instructions
- Women who require better pregnancy protection should at least combine the female condom with a more effective method (not the male latex condom)
- Stress not to wash and reuse a second or third time unless having SI with same partner. New studies demonstrate that this condom may maintain its efficacy for several acts of intercourse. However, reuse is still generally *not* recommended, especially if using to prevent infection. No clinical studies available on the effectiveness after reuse.

CANDIDATES FOR USE: Except for women with pelvic relaxation, any woman may use the female condom. However, the female condom's relatively high cost, difficulty of use, and its high failure rate usually limit its use to women whose partners cannot or will not use a male condom. Specific candidates include:
- Couples willing to accept relatively high failure rates
- Couples who need method directed by woman
- Women needing protection postpartum (if intercourse not uncomfortable)

Special applications for infection control in couples not able to use male condoms:
- Non-monogamous couples (pregnant or not pregnant)
- New couples
- After pregnancy or after pregnancy loss, to reduce risk of endometritis
- Couples with known chronic viral infections (HIV, HPV, HSV) involved in areas sheathed by device

Adolescents: May be offered method, but cost, problems with proper placement and high failure rate detract from its desirability

INITIATING METHOD

- Women planning to use the female condom need to have a chance to study instructions and practice inserting and using method prior to relying on it; 25% in one study could ◄ not insert female condom the first time *[Artz-2002]*
- Patients also benefit from counseling about:
  - How to negotiate with partner to be able to successfully use
  - Need to use with every act of intercourse and how to deal with device mishaps
- In addition, provide ECPs to women relying on female condoms for birth control to ensure immediate use after condom failures. This will minimize risk of unintended pregnancy

INSTRUCTIONS

- Open packaging carefully. Avoid scissors or sharp objects that could cut or tear device
- Patient should rest comfortably in squat or lithotomy position
- Compress inner ring of device and introduce into vagina much like a diaphragm. Use inner ring to guide sheath high into vagina until the outer ring rests against vulva. Rotate inner ring to stabilize device in vault. Avoid tearing condom with fingernails or jewelry. See package instructions for details and drawings illustrating insertion
- Penis should be manually placed (by either man or woman) into the sheath for intercourse and care should be taken to avoid penile contact outside the female condom
- Either woman or man should manually stabilize outer ring against perineum during intercourse to prevent loss of device into the vagina
- Man should monitor for any friction between penis and device which can cause condom breakage or device inversion
- Remove condom immediately after intercourse. Test condom for patency and discard
- If there is any dislocation of the female condom during intercourse or any breakage or spillage of the ejaculate into genitalia, have patient place vaginal spermicide immediately and start her ECPs ASAP. If woman has no ECPs, have her call 1-888-NOT-2-LATE or check www.not-2-late.com/ to locate a provider of ECPs in her area (available through pharmacist in some states). If at risk for STIs when condom fails, seek medical care
- CAUTION: When a latex male condom is used with a polyurethane female condom there ◄ can be an increased risk of breakage of either or both condoms. The oil-based lubricant of the female condom can cause breakage of the male condom. Friction could cause breakage of either

FOLLOW-UP

- Have you had any problems using the female condom?
- Have you had intercourse—even once—without a female condom?
- Do you know how to use ECPs? Do you need more ECPs?
- Do you plan to have children? OR Do you plan to have more children? When?

PROBLEM MANAGEMENT

- Difficulty inserting device: Offer to formally (re)instruct patient
- Problems with removal: Recommend relaxation techniques or have partner remove
- Condom dislodgement or inversion or penis inserted outside condom: Insert a new condom prior to continuing intercourse. Have patient take ECPs if any spill suspected. If at risk for STIs, seek medical care

FERTILITY AFTER USE

- Immediate return to baseline fertility
- Female condom may protect fertility by reducing risk of cervical or vaginal STIs, which can cause upper tract disease and subsequent infertility

DESCRIPTION

Prentif Cavity Rim Cervical Cap is a thimble-shaped latex rubber device with a small groove in its inner surface, which creates suction to keep cap on cervix. Four sizes are available with internal diameters of 22, 25, 28, 31 mm. A small amount of spermicide is placed inside the cap before it is placed over the cervix. When used as a primary method, cervical cap should be coupled with advance prescription of emergency contraceptive pills (ECPs)

EFFECTIVENESS (Rates include use with spermicide cream or jelly)

	Parous	Nulliparous
Perfect use failure rate in first year:	26%	9% ◄
Typical use failure rate in first year:	32%	16% ◄

[Trussell J IN Contraceptive Technology, 2004] (See Table 13.2, p. 38)

MECHANISM

Acts both as a mechanical barrier to sperm migration into the cervical canal and as a chemical agent by applying the spermicide directly to the cervix

ADVANTAGES

Menstrual: None

Sexual/psychological
- Intercourse may be more pleasurable because fear of pregnancy is reduced
- Controlled by the woman
- Can be inserted up to 6 hours prior to sexual intercourse to permit spontaneity in lovemaking
- Can remain in place for multiple acts of sexual intercourse for up to 48 hours total ◄ from time of placement

Cancers, tumors, and masses: None

Other:
- May reduce risk of cervical infections, including gonorrhea, chlamydia and PID
- Immediately active after placement

DISADVANTAGES

Menstrual: None

Sexual/psychological
- Requires placement prior to genital contact, which may reduce spontaneity of sex
- Some women do not like placing fingers or foreign body into vagina

Cancers, tumors, and masses
- Labeling requires repeat Pap smear at 3 months after initiation because increased risk of cervical dysplasia at 3 months; no increase at 1 year. Data submitted to FDA in ◄ follow-up studies shows no increase in dysplasia

Other:
- Lack of protection against some STIs and HIV. Must use condoms if at risk
- Relatively high failure rate, especially in parous women
- Must be refitted postpartum since cervix changes ◄
- Requires professional fitting and requires formal (although brief) training
- About 80% of women can be fitted

- Severe obesity or arthritis may make it difficult for patient to place correctly
- Odor may develop if cap left in place too long, if not appropriately cleansed, or if used during bacterial vaginosis

COMPLICATIONS

- UTIs may increase as coliform counts increase in vagina
- Cervical erosion may occur causing vaginal spotting and/or cervical discomfort. Some women change size of cervix during cycle and need two different size caps
- No cases of toxic shock have been reported, but theoretically, the risk may be increased, particularly if cap were left in for longer than recommended or used during menses
- Allergic reactions to latex may be life threatening; 2-3% of Americans (men and women) have a latex allergy; up to 14% of latex workers are sensitized

CANDIDATES FOR USE

- Women willing and able to insert device prior to coitus and remove it later
- Women with smooth symmetrical cervix which can be fit successfully
- Women with pelvic relaxation are better candidates for cap than for diaphragm
- Women and partner(s) who have no allergies to latex/spermicides

Adolescents: appropriate option, but fitting and insertion may be difficult and offers no protection against certain STIs including HIV. Requires high motivation level

INITIATING METHOD

- Given the high failure rates for the cervical cap, it is very important to provide ECPs ◄— in advance to enable immediate use after cervical cap dislodgement or non-use
- The cervical cap must be professionally fit and refit after each pregnancy ◄—
- A speculum exam is required to judge the size and contour of the cervix, to evaluate for acute cervicitis and vaginitis, and to obtain a Pap smear
- If no nodules, lesions, cysts or other vaginal or cervical abnormalities preclude cap use, a rough estimate is made of the diameter of the cervix
- On bimanual exam, the uterine size and position, and the position, length and diameter of the cervix are determined
- Starting with the smallest likely size cap, squeeze the sides of the rim together and hold the cap with the dome pointing downward
- Apply a small amount of lubricant to the outside edge to facilitate insertion
- With the patient in the lithotomy position, separate her labia and gently insert the cap into the vagina. Guide it into place until the rim slides over the sides of the cervix
- Check for adequate cervical coverage, proper seal and position stability
- The dome of the cap should completely cover the cervix; the rim of the cap tucked snugly and evenly into the fornices; there should be no gap between rim and cervix
- The cap should adhere to the cervix firmly; it should not dislodge during the fitting exam
- To evaluate the fit, make a 360° sweep of the cap rim with the vaginal examining finger to search for gaps or exposed parts of the cervix
- If a gap is found, see if the rim can be pulled away with direct pressure
- After the cap has been in place for at least a minute, check the suction by pinching the excess rubber on the dome between the tips of two fingers and tugging
- The dome should dimple but should not collapse
- Cap should not be dislodged by manual manipulations such as gently pushing and tugging on it with one or two fingers from several angles
- After successful fitting, remove the cap by pushing the rim away from the cervix with one or two fingers to break the suction and then gently pull the cap out of the vagina
- Have patient demonstrate her ability to insert and remove cervical cap

INSTRUCTIONS FOR PATIENT TO USE

- Fill the bottom 1/3 of the inner aspect of the cap with 2% spermicide jelly and put the cap in place prior to sexual intercourse
- Test the fit to insure cervix is covered, sweep with finger 360° around device and check— that there are no gaps between the cervix and the cap; after suction develops for about 1 minute, check that the device does not dislodge with pressure
- Keep the cap in place for 6 hours after last sexual intercourse
- If multiple acts of sexual intercourse occur, there is no need to add more spermicide but do verify correct placement of the device before each episode of sexual intercourse
- Do not use the cap for more than 48 hours at a time, at the time of an infection, or during menses
- Do not expose the cap to petroleum-based products such as vaseline, baby oil, fungicidal creams and petroleum-based antibiotic creams (Listed in figure 18.1, p. 55)
- If cap dislodges, have patient start ECPs ASAP. If woman has no ECPs, have her call 1-888-NOT-2-LATE or check www.not-2-late.com to locate a provider of ECPs in her area. In some states, ECPs are available from a pharmacist without a prescription —
- Use a backup method for first few uses until you are confident in your use of the cap
- Combining the cervical cap and the male condom can increase pregnancy protection and decrease STD transmission
- The FDA recommends a follow-up Pap smear after 3 months
- Do not use cap for at least 2 or 3 days prior to Pap smears

HOW TO REMOVE

- Cap should not be removed until 6 hours after last ejaculation, but prior to 48 hours of use
- Insert a finger into the vagina until the rim of the cap is felt
- Press the cap rim until the seal against the cervix is broken; then tilt the cap off the cervix
- Hook finger around the rim and pull it sideways out of the vagina
- The device must be washed, rinsed, dried and stored in a cool, dark and dry location. Rinsing in Listerine can prevent odors. Corn starch may keep cap dry

FOLLOW-UP

- Are you or your partner experiencing any tenderness or irritation?
- Is the odor of the cap a problem?
- Do you use the cap every single time you have sexual intercourse?
- Do you have any problems with ECPs? Do you need more ECPs?
- Do you plan to have children? OR Do you plan to have more children? If yes, when?

PROBLEM MANAGEMENT

- Allergic reaction to latex: Stop use and switch to another method
- Spotting/cervical tenderness/erosion: Stop use to allow healing; refit with larger cap; rule out STI
- Malodor of device: Listerine soaks may help; shorten time left in place, or replace cap
- Failure to use correctly: Use emergency contraception. If not already available, call 1-888-NOT-2-LATE or check www.not-2-late.com

FERTILITY AFTER USE: Immediate return to baseline fertility

DESCRIPTION: Rubber dome-shaped device filled with spermicide and placed to cover cervix; three types of diaphragms are available:

- Arcing spring: exerts pressure evenly around its rim to cover the cervix
- Coil spring: most appropriate for women with a deep pubic arch with average vaginal tone
- Wide seal: extends inward from the rim to contain the spermicide. Available only through manufacturer
- There are 9 pages of diagrams of diaphragm placement in *A Clinical Guide For Contraception* by Speroff & Darney

EFFECTIVENESS (See Table 13.2, p. 38)
Perfect use failure rate in first year: 6%
Typical use failure rate in first year: 16% ⬅
[Trussell J IN Contraceptive Technology 2004] ⬅

Arcing Spring

MECHANISM

Acts both as a mechanical barrier to sperm migration into the cervical canal and as a spermicide

Coil Spring

ADVANTAGES

Menstrual: None
Sexual/psychological:

- Controlled by the woman
- May be placed by the woman in anticipation of intercourse (within 6 hrs)
- May make sexual intercourse more enjoyable by reducing risk of pregnancy

Wide Seal Rim

Cancers, tumors, and masses: None
Other:

- Reduces risk for cervical STIs, including gonorrhea, chlamydia, cervical dysplasia, and PID (but should not be assumed to be protective against HIV infection)
- Is used only with sexual intercourse
- May be used during lactation after vagina and cervix have achieved non-pregnant shape
- Immediately active after placement

DISADVANTAGES

Menstrual: None
Sexual/psychological:

- Requires placement prior to genital contact which can interrupt spontaneity of sexual intercourse
- Taste of spermicide may discourage certain foreplay activities
- May become messy with multiple acts of intercourse
- Some women dislike placing fingers or foreign bodies into vagina

Cancer, tumors, and masses: None

Other:

- Requires professional fitting; severe obesity may make fitting difficult; must be refitted after pregnancy since cervix changes
- May not be feasible for women with pelvic relaxation
- Requires brief, formal training in use and some dexterity to place and remove device
- May develop odor if not properly cleansed
- Severe obesity or arthritis may make insertion/removal difficult

COMPLICATIONS

- Increases risk of UTI, as result of increase in coliform count in vaginal flora
- May increase risk of TSS, especially if used for prolonged periods or during menses
- Large, poorly fitted diaphragm may cause vaginal erosions

CANDIDATES FOR USE

- Women who can predict when intercourse will occur
- Couples willing to interrupt sex to insert if not done beforehand
- Highly motivated women willing to use with every coital act

Adolescents: Appropriate, if taught to use consistently and correctly; requires discipline

INITIATING METHOD

- Given the high failure rates among users of the diaphragm it is extremely important that clinicians provide women ECPs in advance!
- Needs to be professionally fitted
- Examination with speculum will rule out any vaginal/cervical abnormalities
- On bimanual exam, introduce your third finger into the posterior fornix and tilt your wrist upward to mark where on your index finger/hand contacts the symphysis. Use that measurement as a guide to select the size diaphragm to use and place a fitting diaphragm in the vagina
- Check to ensure diaphragm is lodged behind symphysis and completely covers the cervix. Have patient bear down and visually check to ensure that diaphragm does not move from behind pubic arch
- Have woman walk around for a while in your office to test its long-term comfort
- Have woman demonstrate her ability to insert and remove diaphragm
- Encourage use of a backup method for first few uses to ensure correct use before relying exclusively on diaphragm for protection
- Suggest patient wear diaphragm for 6 hours before using it for contraception to ensure that it is comfortable and can be worn for 6 hours after intercourse

INSTRUCTIONS FOR USE

- Fill inner surface of device 2/3 full with 2 teaspoons of spermicide prior to insertion. It can remain in place for up to 24 hours total from time of placement. Place before genital contact but no longer than 6 hours before coitus

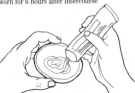

Figure 21.1 Risk of pregnancy increases when a spermicide is not used. Put spermicide on rim and on inside

- Prior to each act of coitus, reconfirm correct placement. For the second and each subsequent act, add additional spermicide vaginally but do not remove the device
- Leave in place for 6 hours after the last act of sexual intercourse ←
- Avoid using any petroleum-based vaginal products such as Vaseline, antifungal creams or some antibiotic creams. (See list of products UNSAFE to use with latex condoms on Figure 18.1, p. 55)
- After removal, clean with soap and water, rinse, dry, and store in the case in a cool, clean, dry, dark area. Corn starch may keep diaphragm dry
- Inspect periodically for any stiffness, holes, cracks, or other defects
- Have it checked each year by a professional. Replace at least every 2 years. Recheck for correct fit whenever there is a 20% weight change and after each pregnancy
- Combine diaphragm with male condoms to reduce pregnancy and STI risk
- If diaphragm dislodges or is not used properly, use EC

Figure 21.2 Reconfirm correct placement of the diaphragm by feeling the cervix through the diaphragm

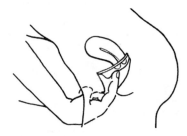

FOLLOW-UP
- Is the diaphragm comfortable? Do you feel excessive pressure?
- Do you get bladder infections often?
- Have you or your partner had an allergic reaction, i.e., burning or itching?
- Do you use the diaphragm consistently? If not, what keeps you from using this method everytime?
- Do you always apply a spermicide prior to insertion?
- Do you have any problems with ECPs? Do you need more ECPs?
- Do you plan to have children? OR Do you plan to have more children? If yes, when?

PROBLEM MANAGEMENT
Prone to cystitis: Urinate postcoitally to reduce bladder colonization with vaginal bacteria; check fit to make sure there is not excessive urethral pressure ←
Allergy to latex: Discontinue use and discuss alternatives. Mylex makes a silicone diaphragm

FERTILITY AFTER USE:
No adverse effects on fertility; may reduce risk of PID. Immediate return to baseline fertility

DESCRIPTION

The search for an effective vaginal microbicide that would also kill sperm remains an important research priority, perhaps the most important research priority, in reproductive health. In the USA, nonoxynol-9 (N-9) is available over the counter. In addition to N-9, patients around the world use menfegol, benzalkonium chloride, sodium docusate, and chlorhexidine. Spermicides are available as vaginal creams, films, foams, gels, suppositories, sponges and tablets.

> A WHO consultation held in Geneva, 9-10 October 2001, concluded that women at high risk of HIV infection should not use products that contain nonoxynol-9. Such women should avoid spermicides containing nonoxynol-9 and nonoxynol-9 lubricated condoms. Condoms without nonoxynol-9 lubrication are effective and widely available. Women at high risk of HIV infection should also avoid using diaphragms and cervical caps to which nonoxynol-9 is added. The contraceptive effectiveness of diaphragms and cervical caps without nonoxynol-9 has been insufficiently studied and should be assumed to be less than that of diaphragms and cervical caps with nonoxynol-9.
>
> ► The Food and Drug Administration has proposed a labeling change for N-9 products that will indicate that these products may actually increase the possibility of acquiring HIV and other STDs from infected partners.

EFFECTIVENESS (See Table 13.2, p. 38)
Perfect use failure rate in first year: 15% ◄━━
Typical use failure rate in first year: 29% ◄━━ *[Trussell J IN Contraceptive Technology, 2004]*

MECHANISM
As barriers, the vehicles prevent sperm from entering the cervical os. As detergents, the chemicals attack the sperm flagella and body, reducing mobility

ADVANTAGES
Menstrual: None
Sexual/psychological:
- Lubrication heightens satisfaction in both partners
- Ease in application (for some women) prior to sexual intercourse
- Either partner can purchase and apply; requires minimal negotiation
- May be used by woman without partner knowing

Cancers, tumors, and masses:
- Possible decrease in HPV transmission may reduce risk of cervical dysplasia and cancer

Other:
- Available over the counter; requires no medical visit
- Inexpensive and easy to use
- Foam is immediately active with placement
- May be used during lactation ◄━━

DISADVANTAGES

Menstrual: None

Sexual/psychological:

- Films and suppository spermicides require 15 minutes for activation, which may interrupt or delay lovemaking
- Either partner must feel comfortable inserting fingers into vagina
- Insertion is not easy for some couples due to embarrassment or reluctance to touch genitalia
- Some forms, e.g., foam, become "messy" during intercourse
- Possible vaginal, oral, and anal irritation can disrupt or preclude sex
- Taste may be unpleasant

Cancers, tumors, and masses: None

Other:

- Current formulations not protective against transmission of HIV, GC or chlamydia (see p. 149 - statement from 2002 CDC STI Treatment Guidelines). Spermicides may, in women having frequent intercourse with multiple partners, enhance transmission of HIV by irritation of vaginal mucosa and by destroying vaginal flora, e.g., lactobacilli, in nonoxynol-9 concentrations as low as 0.1% *[Van Dame, Durban, 2000 found 1.7 RR of HIV transmission in users of spermicidal vaginal gel with 52.5 mg N-9] [Kreiss - 1992]*
- Allergic reactions and dermatitis in women and men that could decrease compliance

COMPLICATIONS

- Women and men have confused fruit jelly, e.g., grape jelly, for spermicidal "jelly"
- Women and men have attempted to use cosmetics or hair products containing non-spermicidal octoxynols and nonoxynols (nonoxynol 4, 10, 12, and 14) in lieu of nonoxynol-9

CANDIDATES FOR USE

- Any woman and partner who presents with no prior allergy or reaction to spermicides

Adolescents:

- Readily available and not contraindicated for teens unless at high risk for HIV infection
- High failure rate may discourage long-term use as primary method

INITIATING METHOD

- Except in cases where the patient, or partner, presents with pregnancy, allergy, or irritation, women can begin these methods at any time following product instructions
- Provide ECPs in advance

INSTRUCTIONS FOR PATIENT

- Before and after applying spermicide, inserting person should wash and dry hands
- Foam spermicide container must have active date and no defects
- Spermicide has its greatest efficacy near the cervical os
- Encourage more spermicide for each act of sexual intercourse
- Water exposure, e.g. bathing or douching, within 6 hours after insertion or post-coitally can minimize effectiveness; reapply before next penetrative act
- Keep spermicides in cool, dry places; tablets or foam can tolerate heat, film melts at 98.6° F

Creams/foams/gels
- Apply less than 1 hour prior to sexual intercourse. May drip out of vagina if inserted more than 1 hour in advance. With foam, shake canister vigorously. Fill plastic applicator with spermicide. Insert applicator deeply into vagina and depress plunger. Immediately active. Finish sexual intercourse within 60 minutes of application

Film, suppositories and tablets
- Insert at least 15 minutes before sexual intercourse: with film, fold the sheet in half and then half again (this aids insertion). Using fingers or an applicator, the inserting partner places the spermicide applicator or film deep in the vagina, near cervix. Finish sexual intercourse within 60 minutes of application

FOLLOW-UP
- Have you or your partner(s) experienced any rash or discomfort after using spermicides?
- Have you changed partners since beginning spermicides?
- Have you had sex—even once—without using spermicides?
- Did you have problems with ECPs?
- Do you need more ECPs?
- Do you plan to have children? OR Do you plan to have more children? If yes, when?

PROBLEM MANAGEMENT
Dermatitis: Discontinue spermicides and offer another method. If vehicle served as lubricant, recommend a water-based or silicone-based lubricant without nonoxynol-9 or octoxynol-9

Changed partners: Explain STI prevention, check for STIs, and recommend condoms

FERTILITY AFTER USE: Immediate return to baseline fertility

WILL THE SPONGE EVER RETURN?
For thousands of years, women have placed sponges with a variety of spermicides into the vagina. We thought that the Today Contraceptive Sponge was going to be back on US pharmacy shelves by the end of 2001. Perhaps this will happen in 2003. Call (201) 934-4449 for further information, to order Today Sponges, and to request educational materials. The company's production plant is awaiting final approval.

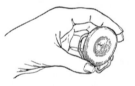

Researchers at University of Texas, Galveston found 3 vaginal lubricants that are safe, non-irritating (unlike nonoxynol-9), and strongly inhibited HIV replication in vitro: Astroglide, Vagisil, and ViAmor. Further studies are needed to determine if they have the same effect in vivo. *[AIDS Research and Human Retroviruses - 2001]*

DESCRIPTION
Man withdraws penis completely from the vagina before ejaculation

EFFECTIVENESS
Perfect use failure rate in first year: 4% (See Table 13.2, p. 38)
Typical use failure rate in first year: 27% ◄
[Trussell J IN Contraceptive Technology, 2004]

MECHANISM
Withdrawal prior to ejaculation reduces or eliminates sperm introduced into vagina.
Preejaculatory fluid is not generally a problem unless two acts of sexual intercourse are close together

COST: None

ADVANTAGES
Menstrual: None
Sexual/psychological:
- No barriers
- Readily available method which encourages male involvement
- Good option for postpartum women ◄
Cancers, tumors, and masses: None
Other: Surprisingly effective if used correctly

DISADVANTAGES
Menstrual: None
Sexual/psychological
- May not be applicable for couples with sexual dysfunction such as premature ejaculation or unpredictable ejaculation
- Requires man's cooperation and instruction
- May reduce sexual pleasure of woman and intensity of orgasm of man
- Encourages "spectatoring" or thinking about what is happening during sexual intercourse
- Limits coital positions (man must be able to withdraw) ◄
Cancers, tumors, and masses: None
Other: **Relatively high failure rate among typical users and does not protect against STIs**

COMPLICATIONS: None

MEDICAL ELIGIBILITY CHECKLIST
- Man must be able to predict ejaculation in time to withdraw penis completely from vagina and move away from woman's external genitalia
- Premature ejaculation makes method less effective
- Appropriate for couples not at risk for STIs

CANDIDATES FOR USE

- Couples who are able to communicate during sexual intercourse
- Disciplined men who can ignore the powerful instinct, urging them to continue thrusting
- Couples in stable, mutually monogamous relationship
- Couples without religious or cultural prohibitions against withdrawal
- Women willing to accept higher risk of unintended pregnancy

Adolescents: Compliance may be a problem (as it is for couples of all ages); teens may have less control over ejaculation; advise use of condoms for better protection against pregnancy and STIs. While withdrawal is a relatively poor contraceptive option, especially if pregnancy prevention and infection control are very important, withdrawal is definitely better than using no contraceptive at all

INITIATING METHOD: Can begin at any time; provide ECPs in advance

INSTRUCTIONS FOR PATIENT

- Practice withdrawal using backup method until both partners master withdrawal
- Wipe penis clean of the pre-ejaculation fluid prior to vaginal penetration
- Use coital positions that ensure that the man will be capable of withdrawing easily at ◄— the appropriate time
- Use emergency contraception if withdrawal fails

FOLLOW-UP

- Do your partner(s) ever ejaculate/begin to ejaculate before withdrawing?
- Did you have any problems with ECPs? Do you need more ECPs?
- Do you plan to have children? OR Do you plan to have more children?

PROBLEM MANAGEMENT

Failure to withdraw: Use ECPs if withdrawal does not occur every time. Consider another method

FERTILITY AFTER USE: No adverse effects on fertility

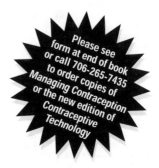

Please see form at end of book or call 706-265-7435 to order copies of Managing Contraception or the new edition of Contraceptive Technology

OVERVIEW

Emergency contraception (EC) includes any method that acts after intercourse to *prevent pregnancy*. None of the current methods is an abortifacient and none disturbs an implanted pregnancy. There are currently 3 methods in widespread use worldwide:

- High-dose progestin-only contraceptive pills (POPs). PLAN B preferable to Ovrette or Preven
- (Yuzpe Method) 13 brands of combined oral contraceptive pills (COCs). PREVEN preferable to other COCs as package insert describes use as an EC; Preven may be more expensive
- Copper IUD insertion (Paragard)

An estimated 51,000 pregnancies were averted by EC use in 2000 accounting for 43% of the ◄— decrease in abortions since 1994 *[Finer-2003]*. Only the two hormonal methods are utilized to any significant degree in the U.S. (all combined and progestin-only pills that may be used are on p. 78 of this book and in colored diagram on A-24). Provide to patients in advance in one of 2 ways: give them pills in advance or give them a prescription with refills in advance

Table 24.1 Overview of Postcoital Methods Currently Available in U.S.

Characteristic	POPs	COCs *	Copper IUD
Timing of initiation after intercourse	ASAP but *can* be used up to 120 hours (5 days) ◄— Sooner is better	ASAP but *can* be used on days 4 & 5 after unprotected sex; Sooner is better	Up to 8 days
Pregnancies/ 100 women	Early start: 0.4% (<12 h) Late start: 2.7% (1-3 days) Average: 1.1%	Early start: 0.5% (<12 h) Late start: 4.2% (1-3 days) Average: 2 - 3.2%	0.1%
Advantages	Fewer side effects than Preven or COCs; Product available for advance prescription: Plan B®	Product available for advance prescription: PREVEN™; Wide range of COCs available for use	May be inserted 5 or more days after intercourse, but before implantation. Effective long-term contraceptive for appropriate women
Disadvantages	Less available than COCs that can be used to create an off-label EC regimen. Check for availability of Plan B at pharmacies near you at www.go2planb.com	Gastrointestinal side effects – can be reduced with antiemetic pretreatment	Expensive; must be appropriate candidate for IUD; Timing issues: counseling, testing, etc. Insertion procedure required
Side effects	Spotting. Same hormonal side effects as COCs, but less frequent and less severe	Nausea, vomiting, spotting headache, breast tenderness, moodiness, change in next menses	Pain, bleeding, expulsion
Avoid use in pregnant women and women with other prescribing precautions	Do not use in women with known pregnancy because the treatment will not be effective. Not teratogen	Do not use in women with known pregnancy or current severe migraine. POPs a better option for all women history of DVT or PE	Prescribing precautions for IUD use (see page 80)

For more information about EC, phone numbers of EC providers, or **to become listed as an EC provider**, check out the web site www.not-2-late.com or call the EC Hotline at 1-888-NOT-2-LATE. Other good sources of information about EC are www.preven.com or 1-888-PREVEN-2 and www.go2planb.com or call 800-330-1271.

* COCs using norgestrel are better studied, but COCs with norethindrone may be used as ECPs, but ◄— failure rates are slightly higher

EMERGENCY CONTRACEPTION WITH EMERGENCY CONTRACEPTIVE PILLS

DESCRIPTION

POPs: more effective than COCs and less side effects ◀—

- Research indicates both tablets can be taken together in a single dose without significant reduction in efficacy or increase in side effects ◀—
- ➤ Both Plan B tabs or 1.5 mg of norgestrel at once OR in divided doses, take first dose ASAP within 120 hours after inadequately protected sex; take second dose 12-24 hours later (second dose may be more than 120 hours after unprotected sex).
  Second dose may also be taken less than 12 hours after the first dose ◀—
- Plan B is the only currently-available FDA-approved progestin-only product with instructions and pills that facilitate advance prescription
- Ovrette (20 yellow pills for each dose; she needs 2 packs of Ovrette)

Yuzpe Method using any of the levonorgestrel-containing COCs:

- Two large doses of COCs with at least 100 μg of ethinyl estradiol and either 100 mg of norgestrel or 50 mg of levonorgestrel. Take first dose ASAP within 72 hours after inadequately protected sex; take second dose 12 hours later (second dose may be taken up to 120 hours after unprotected sex). Try to provide ECPs to women in advance (actual pills or prescription with refills) (see Figure 24.1, p. 78)
- The Preven™ Emergency Contraceptive Kit facilitates utilizing combined OCs

EFFECTIVENESS: A randomized WHO trial of two levonorgestrel regimens (using LNg pills that were the same as Plan B tablets) found that taking 2 Plan B tablets at once was as effective (failure rate 1.5%) as taking 1 Plan B tablet followed by a second in 12 hours (failure rate 1.8%). The levonorgestrel dose need NOT be split. Both Plan B tablets may be taken at once without an increase in nausea (15%) or vomiting (1%). In this large trial, starting treatment with a delay of 4-5 days did not significantly increase the failure rate compared to the efficacy of treatment begun within 3 days of unprotected intercourse. *[von Hertzen 2002].* Failure rate was slightly higher but not significantly higher when ECPs were taken on days 4 or 5

EC with POPs PLAN B	Only 1.1% of 967 women using POPs for EC became pregnant in a WHO multi-center study *[WHO task force on Postovulatory Methods of Fertility Regulation. Lancet Aug 8, 1998]*	89% average reduction of pregnancy rate based on WHO perfect-use study population	12 pregnancies per 1000 unprotected acts of sexual intercourse followed by Plan B
EC with COCs Preven	2-3% failure rate	74% average reduction of pregnancy rate (WHO perfect-use study)	20-32 pregnancies per 1000 unprotected acts of sexual intercourse followed by Preven or COCs

- Taking more than number of pills specified is *not* beneficial (unless patient is taking medications such as anticonvulsants or St. John's Wort that require higher doses of EC) and may increase risk of vomiting ◀—

MECHANISMS

- ECPs act by preventing pregnancy and never by disrupting an implanted pregnancy, i.e. never as an abortifacient
- If taken before ovulation, ECPs disrupt normal follicular development and maturation, blocks LH surge, and inhibit ovulation; they may also create deficient luteal phase and may have a contraceptive effect by thickening cervical mucus
- If taken after ovulation, ECPs have little effect on ovarian hormonal production and limited effect on endometrial maturation

72• ECPs may affect tubal transport of sperm or ova

COST

POPs:

- Plan B is available in selected retail pharmacies for about $25. To find a pharmacy check out www.go2planb.com
- Ovrette (2 packs) is not readily available in all pharmacies and can cost up to $70
- Non-profit and Title X agencies may purchase Plan B at $4.50 - $8.00 per treatment ◄──
- Pharmacists in those states that may dispense without a prescription charge $50-$55 ◄── for counseling and medication

Yuzpe method with COCs:

- The Preven™ kit: Pills plus pregnancy test: $20-$25 at some retail pharmacies. Publicly supported clinics can buy Preven™ kit less expensively (without pregnancy test) ◄──
- One cycle of COCs may vary from a few dollars to more than $50.

Other costs:

- Cost prior to obtaining pills may vary from nothing (if already given) to cost of full exam and pregnancy test

ADVANTAGES

Menstrual: None

Sexual/Psychological:

- Offers an opportunity to prevent pregnancy after rape, mistake, or overt barrier method failure (condom breaks or slips, diaphragm dislodges, etc.)
- Reduces anxiety about unintended pregnancy prior to next menses
- Process of getting EC may lead woman to initiate ongoing contraception

Cancers, tumors and masses: None

Other:

- There are 3 million unintended pregnancies each year; nearly half of all pregnancies are unintended. *[Henshaw, 1998]* Widespread availability of ECPs could halve the number of unintended pregnancies and the consequent need for abortion *[Trussell, 1992]*
- 40% of reduction in teen pregnancies ('95 to '99) due to EC ◄──
- Could reduce birth defects (poor use of folic acid if conception is not planned)
- Reduces ectopic pregnancy rate

DISADVANTAGES

Menstrual:

- Next menses may be early (especially if taken before ovulation), on time, or late
- Notable changes in flow of next menses seen in 10-15% of women
- **If no menses within 3 weeks (21 days) of taking ECPs, pregnancy test should be done** ◄──

Sexual/psychological:

- Women who are uncomfortable with post-fertilization methods might need reassurance that use of EC with COCs or POPs is consistent with their beliefs if taken during the follicular phase. They also may need to be warned that if taken after ovulation, ECPs may work as an interceptive (ie prevent implantation of fertilized egg)

Cancers, tumors and masses: None

Other:

- Breast tenderness, fatigue, headache, abdominal pain and dizziness
- No protection against STIs; consider treatment for possible STIs following exposure

Nausea and vomiting:

	Nausea	Vomiting	Pretreatment with antiemetic
POPs	23%	6%	Needed only if Hx of past problems
COCs	50%	19%	Can reduce symptoms by 30-50%

COMPLICATIONS

• Several cases of DVT reported in women using COCs as ECPs. No increased DVT risk with POPs

CANDIDATES FOR USE: Definitely can be given to men ←

• All women who have had or who may be at risk for unprotected sex (sperm exposure) are candidates for ECPs for immediate or future use. Women with strong contraindications to estrogen use should use POPs (see PRESCRIBING PRECAUTIONS)
• As a backup method for less effective barrier methods ←
• There are many situations in which women have unintended sperm exposure:
  • Failed contraceptive methods: broken condom, dislodged diaphragm, or cervical cap, ←
    forgotten pills, late for contraceptive reinjection, NFP miscalculation, failed withdrawal
  • Failure to use methods: clouded judgment, passion, sexual assault
• For the woman who has intercourse infrequently (1-2x/yr) Particularly effective if ←
  taken within one hour of otherwise unprotected sex
• Note: ECPs do not protect as well as ongoing methods
Adolescents: appropriate back-up option (consider providing ECPs in advance)

PRECAUTIONS

Labeling for Plan B lists only 3 prescribing precautions:
• Pregnancy (no benefit; no effect)
• Hypersensitivity to any component of product
• Undiagnosed abnormal vaginal bleeding

Labeling for Preven (and for all COCs used for EC) lists a wide range of contraindications inherited from the labeling for COCs. In reality, use of COCs should be allowed for all women except those who:
• Are pregnant; no benefit but also no dangers
• Are known to be hypersensitive to any component of the product
• Have acute migraine headaches at the time ECPs are to be taken (Use Plan B)
• Have history of DVT or PE (use POPs - Plan B)

INITIATING METHOD: Pregnancy testing is *optional*, not required:

• Offer ECPs routinely to all women who may be at risk for unprotected intercourse
  • Advance prescription increases use of EC but does not diminish use of primary method of contraception
  • Availability directly through pharmacists led to a thousand-fold increase in use of ECPs in selected pharmacies in the state of Washington
  • Self-contained kits such as Preven and Plan B, which come with FDA-approved instructions, are more likely to be taken correctly than off-label regimens. A study at the University of Pennsylvania found that women given a full packet of Nordette followed a variety of regimens from 1 tablet a day for 21 days (wrong!) to 21 tablets in a day (wrong!)
• Provide EC for all women who present after-the-fact, acutely in need. If you dispense off-label pills in your clinic, be sure to have her remove the inactive pills to reduce risk of mistake
• Patient history for prescribing EC after-the-fact:
  • LMP, previous menstrual period, dates of any prior unprotected intercourse this cycle, and date and time of last unprotected intercourse
  • Any problems with previous use of ECPs, COCs or POPs?
  • Breast-feeding or severe headaches now? History of DVT or PE? (Use POPs rather than COCs)
  • Any foreseeable problems if antiemetic causes drowsiness?

- No physical exam/labs needed on a routine basis:
  - No pelvic exam is necessary, now or in the past; No BP measurements needed
  - Pregnancy testing useful <u>only</u> if concerned that prior intercourse may have caused pregnancy. *ACOG, IPPF and WHO do not include routine pregnancy testing in their protocols*
- Advise patient about possible side effects and consider other EC options (Copper IUD)
- If prescribing Preven, premedicate with long-acting antiemetic one hour prior to first ECP dose. Take two tablets of meclizine hydrochloride 25 mg (over-the-counter Dramamine II or Bonine). Other agents work, but do not have same duration of action. Avoid antiemetic if drowsiness will pose safety hazard. Antiemetics not needed prior to Plan B
- Offer appropriate number of tablets for particular ECP brand to reach adequate dose (see Figure 24.1, p.78 and p. A-26 opposite inside back cover)
- Encourage patient to take first dose ASAP and second dose approximately 12 hours after first dose. It is ok to take second dose in slightly less or more than 12 hours; realize that 72 hours is not the absolute limit. Both Plan B tabs may be taken at once ◄——
- Consider providing EC now for patient to have available at home in case she has another need to use EC again OR provide prescription with refills
- Inquire about desire to be checked for STI's (especially in cases of rape) ◄——

STARTING REGULAR USE OF CONTRACEPTIVE AFTER USE OF ECPs

- Start using regular method immediately. ECPs offer no lingering reliable protection
- If missed OCs, restart day after ECPs taken (no need to catch up missed pills)
- If starting COCs, patch or ring, see COC precautions and then:
  - May wait for next menses or
  - Start OCs, patch or ring next day with 7-day backup method (this will affect timing of next menses). In office you may punch out a few pills at the beginning of a pill pack ◄—— to correspond with the date you are seeing her. This will reduce confusion
- If starting DMPA or Lunelle injections, can start immediately. If so, consider having patient return in 2-3 weeks for pregnancy test
- If starting barrier methods, start immediately.
- If starting NFP, use abstinence (or barrier/spermicide) until next menses

SPECIAL ISSUES/FREQUENT QUESTIONS

- When in cycle should EC be offered? Anytime except perhaps if she is having her menses
- How many times a year can a woman use ECPs? No limit
- What if a patient has had unprotected intercourse earlier in the cycle? Do urine test to confirm no obvious pregnancy. Offer EC. If concerned that your test may miss an early ◄—— pregnancy, give EC and have her return in 3 weeks (if no menses) for another pregnancy test. EC will not adversely affect the fetus or a pregnancy
- What if she used EC earlier in the month? Offer it again; she may have just delayed ovulation. Review why her primary contraceptive is failing her and remedy the situation (perhaps with a new method). Consider performing pregnancy test in this setting even though it may be too early to have become positive; counsel her about this possibility
- What if the pharmacy is closed or does not carry EC? Plan ahead—provide EC by advance prescription. Check with local 24-hour pharmacies; encourage stocking up with Plan B. ◄—— Also visit www.go2planb.com
- What if a woman whom I have not seen previously calls for ECPs? Many practitioners screen over the telephone and telephone in prescriptions to pharmacies. In some states, the law requires face to face contact to establish physician-patient relationship

INSTRUCTIONS FOR PATIENT

- For advance prescriptions, advise woman who is using ECPs containing estrogen to purchase long-lasting antiemetic and keep it next to ECPs

- Make sure woman using antiemetic with COCs understands risk of drowsiness. Have her take antiemetic as soon as possible after unprotected sexual intercourse
- Wait 12 hours, then take second dose of ECPs (Second dose of antiemetic unnecessary if long-acting antiemetic was used). Both doses of Plan B may be taken at once ←
- Start using protection right away. ECPs do not reliably protect you beyond the day they are used
- Return for pregnancy testing if she has not had her menses 21 days after using ECPs
- Re-evaluate primary contraceptive method to make it more reliable

FOLLOW-UP
- No routine follow-up needed
- Have patient return for pregnancy testing if no menses in 3 weeks

PROBLEM MANAGEMENT
Nausea/vomiting:
- In general, POPs are preferable because they are more effective and have lower risk of complications and side effects
- Antiemetic may be prescribed before or after taking combined COCs as ECPs (does not work as well when taken late)
- Vomiting that occurs due to ECPs probably indicates that enough hormones reached the bloodstream to have the desired contraceptive effect. Most experts (but NOT all) recommend a repeat dose of ECPs if vomiting occurs within 30 minutes of taking ECPs. ACOG recommends a repeat dose if vomiting occurs within one hour *[ACOG 1996]*
- If repeating dose because of severe vomiting, switch from COCs to POPs or consider placing pills in vagina rather than mouth (off-label). Although uptake is slower, this may also be possible for woman who has experienced extreme nausea while taking COCs in the past as her regular contraceptive. No data on effectiveness of vaginal COCs used as EC
- If severe vomiting occurs, consider IUD as EC

Amenorrhea:
- If menses do not occur in 21 days (or more than 7 days beyond expected day for menses to begin), need to rule out pregnancy

Pregnancy in spite of using ECPs:
- If there is a pregnancy, the woman should be reassured that there is evidence that ECPs do not increase the risk of fetal anomalies or miscarriage

FERTILITY AFTER USE
Excellent. Fertility returns after next menses (maybe before!)

EMERGENCY CONTRACEPTION WITH COPPER IUD

DESCRIPTION
- Insert Copper IUD, following the usual procedures, within 5 days after unprotected or inadequately protected sexual intercourse. May be used up to 8 days after intercourse, if ovulation is known to have occurred 3 days or more after the unprotected sex
- More frequently used overseas, where IUD costs are lower
- In the US, this method is generally restricted to use by women who intend to continue to use the IUD as an ongoing method; the choice should be the patient's
- Levonorgestrel IUD (Mirena) is NOT indicated for use as EC ←

EFFECTIVENESS
• Failure rate < 1% (only about 6 pregnancies per 1000 insertions in world's literature)

MECHANISMS
• Usually functions as interceptive (after fertilization, but prior to implantation) by interfering with implantation
• Rarely, may act as contraceptive, if inserted days before ovulation

COST
• Expensive (about $500) unless used as a long-term contraceptive method after insertion as EC (see Chapter 25, p. 80-86). In Europe postcoital IUD insertion costs just $25 (Belgium) or is covered by health plan

ADVANTAGES
• The most effective post-coital method
• May be used 2-5 days later than ECPs
• Provides long-term protection against pregnancy following insertion

DISADVANTAGES: Same as using Copper IUD as contraceptive (See Chapter 25, p. 80-86)
• Very expensive, if only used for EC and removal expected soon
• Timing constraints of EC use may make it difficult to properly screen patients for IUD insertion (counseling, preinsertion cultures, etc.)

COMPLICATIONS, CANDIDATES FOR USE, PRESCRIBING PRECAUTIONS, INITIATING METHOD, INSTRUCTIONS FOR PATIENT FOLLOW-UP, PROBLEM MANAGEMENT, FERTILITY AFTER USE
• Same as using Copper IUD as ongoing contraceptive (See Chapter 25, p. 80-86)

EMERGENCY CONTRACEPTION WITH MIFEPRISTONE (RU-486)

DESCRIPTION
• Single 10 mg to 25 mg dose of the anti-progestogen mifepristone (RU-486), taken within 5 days of unprotected intercourse. Not available in the United States. Still not approved by any major regulatory agency in the world

NOT AVAILABLE AS EC FOR WOMEN IN THE U.S.

EFFECTIVENESS
• About the same effectiveness as levonorgestrel (Plan B) in most recent study ←
  Lancet-12/7/02]
• One international study allowed initiation up to 120 hours and still found 85% overall efficacy

MECHANISMS
• Blocks action of progesterone by binding to its receptors
• Stops ovulation if given in follicular phase (contraceptive)
• Slows endometrial maturation in luteal phase (interceptive)

FERTILITY AFTER USE
• Fertility may return later in cycle or with next menses

Figure 24.1

EMERGENCY CONTRACEPTION USING EMERGENCY CONTRACEPTIVE PILLS (ECPs)

1-888-NOT-2 LATE; www.opr.princeton.edu/ec; www.go2planB.com ◄

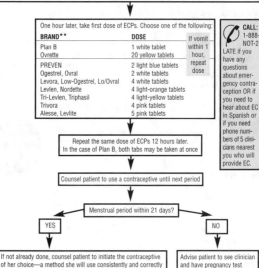

Consider dispensing emergency contraceptive pills (ECPs) (or a prescription for ECPs) **prior to the need** for them so that women and men have them available at home (or rapid access to them) in case they are needed. This is particularly important since some pharmacies will not dispense ECPs

Start ECPs as soon as possible, after unprotected or inadequately protected sexual intercourse. **Can be used up to 5 days, but sooner is better; most effective within 24 hours**

If using PREVEN or another COC, first, take anti-nausea medication: 50 mg oral meclizine* has 24-hour duration of action. No need to use anti-nausea medication if using Plan B

One hour later, take first dose of ECPs. Choose one of the following:

BRAND**	DOSE	
Plan B	1 white tablet	If vomit within 1 hour, repeat dose
Ovrette	20 yellow tablets	
PREVEN	2 light blue tablets	
Ogestrel, Ovral	2 white tablets	
Levora, Low-Ogestrel, Lo/Ovral	4 white tablets	
Levlen, Nordette	4 light-orange tablets	
Tri-Levlen, Triphasil	4 light-yellow tablets	
Trivora	4 pink tablets	
Alesse, Levlite	5 pink tablets	

CALL: 1-888-NOT-2 LATE if you have any questions about emergency contraception OR if you need to hear about EC in Spanish or if you need phone numbers of 5 clinicians nearest you who will provide EC.

Repeat the same dose of ECPs 12 hours later. In the case of Plan B, both tabs may be taken at once

Counsel patient to use a contraceptive until next period

Menstrual period within 21 days?

YES → If not already done, counsel patient to initiate the contraceptive of her choice—a method she will use consistently and correctly

NO → Advise patient to see clinician and have pregnancy test

NOTE: if anti-nausea medication is NOT taken prior to first dose of ECPs (which is recommended), it may be taken after the first dose, though nausea may be severe or should vomit. Anti-nausea medication is usually not needed for women using PLAN B, as PLAN B does not contain estrogen

* Meclizine hydrochloride is recommended because it has a 24-hour duration of action. It is available over the counter as Bonine and as Dramamine 2. If prescribing an antiemetic, use Antivert®. Other medications to prevent nausea may be prescribed instead.

**Norethindrone pills recently shown to be effective

Figure 24.2

EMERGENCY CONTRACEPTION USING COPPER IUD
www.opr.princeton.edu/ec ◄──

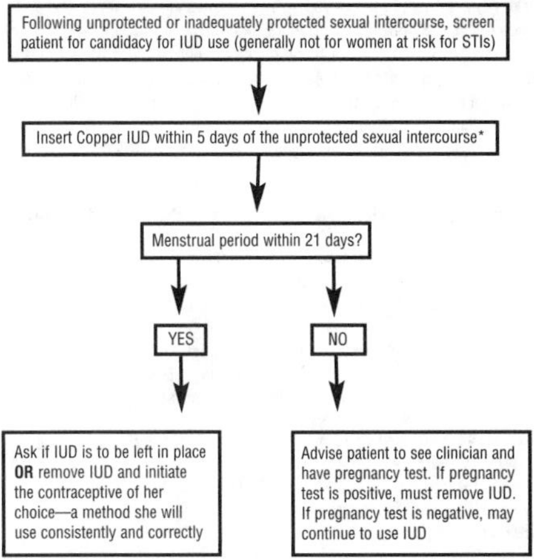

Following unprotected or inadequately protected sexual intercourse, screen patient for candidacy for IUD use (generally not for women at risk for STIs)

Insert Copper IUD within 5 days of the unprotected sexual intercourse*

Menstrual period within 21 days?

YES | NO

Ask if IUD is to be left in place **OR** remove IUD and initiate the contraceptive of her choice—a method she will use consistently and correctly

Advise patient to see clinician and have pregnancy test. If pregnancy test is positive, must remove IUD. If pregnancy test is negative, may continue to use IUD

* The Copper IUD may be inserted up to the time of implantation—about 5 days after ovulation—to prevent pregnancy. Thus, if a woman had unprotected sexual intercourse 3 days before ovulation occurred in that cycle, the IUD could be inserted up to 8 days after intercourse to prevent pregnancy

> **CALL:** 1-888-NOT-2 LATE if you have any questions about emergency contraception OR if you need to hear about EC in Spanish or if you need phone numbers of 5 clinicians nearest you who will provide EC.

OVERVIEW: A Johns Hopkins webpage has pictures of many IUDs. Go to www.jhuccp.org/pr/b6/b6used.stm The only two intrauterine contraceptives available in the U.S. are the ParaGard® T 380A Intrauterine Copper (Copper IUD) and the Mirena® levonorgestrel- releasing intrauterine system (LNG-IUS). The Progestasert System (proges-terone IUD) is no longer marketed in the United States. For intrauterine contraception to play the role it could play, clinicians must become more supportive of the role of insertion immediately following delivery of the placenta. IUDs may also be inserted immediately after an abortion

INTRAUTERINE COPPER CONTRACEPTIVE (ParaGard T 380A)

DESCRIPTION: T-shaped intrauterine contraceptive made of radiopaque polyethylene, with two flexible arms that bend down for insertion but open in the uterus to hold solid sleeves of copper against fundus. Fine copper wire wrapped around stem. Surface area of copper = 380 mm^2. Monofilament polyethylene tail string threaded through and knotted below blunt ball at base of stem creates double strings that protrude into vagina. For medical information: 1-800-682-6532. This IUD has 2 straw colored strings

EFFECTIVENESS *[Trussell J IN Contraceptive Technology, 2004]*
• Approved for 10 years use; effective for at least 12 years
Perfect use failure rate in first year: 0.6% (see Table 13.2, p. 38)
Typical use failure rate in first year: 0.8%
Cumulative 10-year failure rate: 2.1-2.8%

MECHANISMS

The intrauterine copper contraceptive works primarily as a spermicide. Copper ions inhibit sperm motility and acrosomal enzyme activation so that sperm rarely reach the tube and are unable to fertilize the ovum. The sterile inflammatory reaction created in the endometrium phagocytizes the sperm. Experimental evidence suggests that the IUDs do not routinely work after fertilization. They are not abortifacients. They primarily prevent pregnancy by preventing fertilization

COST: From $0 to well over $500
Special Cost Savings Programs: For full-pay purchasers of this IUD: 1-800-322-4966
• 3-month warranty. Manufacturer offers to replace any unit that is lost or must be removed within the first 3 months of use
• Professional courtesy program: any staff member or relative of provider is eligible for a free IUD
• **Manufacturer offers free IUD to patients experiencing financial problems who would otherwise not be able to afford an IUD if the provider will insert it free of charge. Forms are available from Ortho-McNeil representative**

ADVANTAGES: Effective long-term contraception from a single decision

Menstrual: none

Sexual/psychological
- Convenient; permits spontaneous sexual activities. Requires no action at time of use
- Intercourse may be more pleasurable with risk of pregnancy reduced

Cancers, tumors and masses
- Possible protection against endometrial cancer (case control studies)

Other
- Rapid return to fertility and private
- Convenient - single insertion provides up to 12 years protection (package labeling says 10 years)
- **Cost effective. Provides greatest net benefits of any contraceptive over a 5 year period. Every copper IUD inserted saves the health care system $14,133 in its first 5 years of use**
- Good option for women who cannot use hormonal methods
- Risk for ectopic pregnancy decreased 10-fold
- **IUDs lead to highest level of user satisfaction, 95%, of any contraceptive currently being used by women**

DISADVANTAGES

Menstrual
- Average monthly blood loss increased by about 35%; this may be diminished by NSAIDs
- May increase dysmenorrhea (removal rates for bleeding and pain first year = 11.9%)
- Spotting and cramping with insertion and intermittently in weeks following insertion

Sexual/psychological
- Some women uncomfortable with concept of having "something" (foreign body) placed inside them
- Some women are not at ease checking strings
- Strings palpable; if strings cut too short, may cause partner discomfort

Cancers, tumors and masses: None

Other
- Requires office procedure for insertion and removal; both can be uncomfortable
- Some programs/protocols recommend a chlamydia/gc check before insertion, others do not
- Increases risk of infection in first 20 days after insertion (1/1000 women will get PID)
- Offers no protection from HIV/STIs; PID: see data in box below
- May be expelled obviously (with cramping and bleeding) or silently (unknowingly placing woman at risk for pregnancy). Rate of expulsion declines over time. At 5 years cumulative expulsion rate is 11.3%. Expulsion rate for the 5th year is 0.3%

COMPLICATIONS: See PROBLEM MANAGEMENT section for details

Complication	Frequency	Risk factors
PID within 20 days	1/1000	BV, cervicitis, contamination with insertion
Uterine perforation	1/1000	Immobile, markedly verted uterus Breast-feeding woman Inexperienced, unskilled inserter
Vasovagal reaction or Fainting with insertion	Rare	Stenotic os, pain Prior vasovagal reaction
Expulsion		Insertion on menses, too soon postpartum, not high enough in fundus or nulliparous
Pregnancy		Poor placement, expulsion

- Women wanting long-term contraception but wanting to avoid tubal sterilization or poor surgical candidates ◄—
- Currently recommended patient profile includes women in stable mutually monogamous relationships (at low risk of STIs). The copper IUD and LNg IUD are best for women seeking longer-term (≥ 2 years) pregnancy protection due to its initial cost.
- Nulliparous women at low risk for STIs may also be candidates. Nulliparous women with history of PID may be candidates if they are currently in stable mutually monogamous relationships with an uninfected partner and have had a pregnancy since the PID episode
- Good option for women who cannot or do not want to use hormones:
  - Women with personal risk of thrombosis; Breastfeeding women; Smokers over 35; Women who fear hormonal side effects

Adolescents: Adolescents usually do not meet all the criteria for IUD use and may not tolerate increased bleeding and cramping with menses caused by the Copper IUD

PRESCRIBING PRECAUTIONS: See WHO Eligibility Criteria, **pages A1-A8** ◄—
- Pregnancy
- Women with current STI, STI within 3 months or women at risk (multiple sex partners) ◄—
- Uterus < 6 cm or > 9 cm
- Undiagnosed abnormal vaginal bleeding
- Active cervicitis or active pelvic infection or known symptomatic actinomycosis
- Recent endometritis (last 3 months); See WHO recommendations, A-6
- Allergy to copper; Wilson's disease
- Uterine distortion or pathology preventing even distribution of copper ions or fundal placement of IUD
- AIDS (WHO: 3), HIV (WHO: 3) - because women with HIV/AIDS may still be at risk for other ◄— STI's. However, IUD's do not increase complications in women with HIV/AIDS *[Curtis - 2002]* This "3" is not evidence-based ◄—
- Known or suspected uterine or cervical cancer; unresolved abnormal Pap smear
- Severe anemia (relative contraindication) (Levonorgestrel IUD would be a good choice)
- Nulliparous women with small uterus (< 6.0 cm) or at high risk for STIs ◄—

INITIATING METHOD
- Requires insertion by trained professional
- May be inserted at any time in cycle when pregnancy can be ruled out; lowest overall rates of removal are when insertion is at midcycle
- Early expulsion rates lower if avoid insertion during menses
- May be inserted immediately after induced, therapeutic or first trimester spontaneous abortion if infection can be ruled out ◄—
- May be inserted immediately after delivery of the placenta or prior to discharge from hospital after delivery or may await complete uterine involution postpartum or following second or third trimester loss
- One IUD may be removed and a second inserted at the same visit
- Test for cervical infection, if indicated. Rule out BV (treat prior to insertion)

INSERTION TIPS: *Each step should be performed slowly and gently*
- All clinicians wanting to insert IUDs would benefit from training in IUD insertion
- Reconfirm formal consent; Give NSAIDs one hour prior to insertion
- Be sure patient is not pregnant
- Routine antibiotic prophylaxis is not warranted; AHA requires **no** antibiotic treatment for women at risk for bacterial endocarditis
- Recheck position, size and mobility of uterus prior to insertion
- Collect specimens for infection tests, if not done prior to insertion (including vaginal wet mount)

- Cleanse upper vaginal, outer cervix, and cervical os and canal thoroughly with antiseptic
- In some instances provide cervical anesthesia with paracervical block and 1/2 cc lidocaine injected into tenaculum site
- Place tenaculum to stabilize cervix and straighten uterine axis
- Sound uterus to fundus with uterine sound or pipelle; hold sound like a pencil when entering internal os to limit uterine perforation risk
- See Figure 25.1 below for copper IUD insertion directions
- Trim strings to about 2" (5 cm) and tuck around cervix. Avoid cutting strings too short or too long. Some clinicians trim strings to 1 - 1.5" (3-4 cm). Mark length of strings on ⟵ chart for later follow-up visits to confirm that length is the same

Figure 25.1 How to insert a Copper IUD

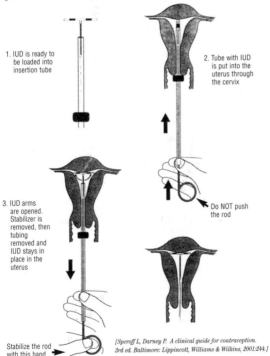

1. IUD is ready to be loaded into insertion tube

2. Tube with IUD is put into the uterus through the cervix

Do NOT push the rod

3. IUD arms are opened. Stabilizer is removed, then tubing removed and IUD stays in place in the uterus

Stabilize the rod with this hand ⟶

[Speroff L, Darney P. A clinical guide for contraception. 3rd ed. Baltimore: Lippincott, Williams & Wilkins, 2001:244.]

POSTPLACENTAL & IMMEDIATE POSTPARTUM INSERTION

- Postplacental (preferably within 10 minutes after expulsion of the placenta) and immediate postpartum insertion during the first week after delivery (but preferably within 48 hours) are convenient effective and safe times to insert copper IUDs
- Expulsion rates of 7-15% at 6 months require that women receiving an IUD very soon after delivery be told how to detect expulsions and instructed to return for reinsertion
- Unplanned pregnancy rates of post placental IUD insertion range from 2.0 - 2.8 per 100 users at 24 months. [O'Hanley, 1992]
- Although service providers find post placental and immediate postpartum insertion *easier* than interval insertion, Engender Health policy states that any clinician interested in learning these techniques needs to receive hands-on training in advance.

> **Figure 25.2 Two techniques of postplacental IUD insertion and proper location of IUD after insertion**

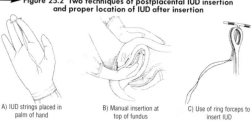

A) IUD strings placed in palm of hand

B) Manual insertion at top of fundus

C) Use of ring forceps to insert IUD

INSTRUCTIONS FOR PATIENT

- Give patient trimmed IUD strings to learn what to check for after menses each month
- Advise patients to return if any symptoms of pregnancy, infection or IUD loss develop:

PAINS: "Early IUD/IUC/IUS Warning Signs"	
P	Period late (pregnancy); abnormal spotting or bleeding
A	Abdominal pain, pain with intercourse
I	Infection exposure (STI); abnormal vaginal discharge
N	Not feeling well, fever, chills
S	String missing, shorter or longer

- Counsel patient on anticipated menstrual changes. Take NSAIDs prophylactically for first 2-3 days of next 3 menses (eg, Ibuprofen 200-400 mg orally every 4-6 hours starting at beginning of menstrual flow). Contact provider if bleeding bothersome

FOLLOW-UP

- Have patient return for post insertion check about 2 1/2 months after insertion to rule out partial expulsion or other problems requiring removal (before end of 3 month warranty). Many clinicians prefer 1 month return visit and then at 2.5 months if any problems.
- Routine annual well-woman exams

FOLLOW-UP CHECKLIST- *Questions to ask women using IUD on each return visit:*

- Do you have any questions about/or problems with your IUD? (Remember PAINS)
- Can you feel your IUD strings? Have they changed in length?
- Have you or your partner had any new partners since your last visit?
- Do you plan to have children? OR Do you plan to have more children? If yes, when?

PROBLEM MANAGEMENT

Uterine perforation:
- All perforations occur at insertion
- Clinical signs: pain, loss of resistance to advancement of instrument and instrument introduced deeper than uterus thought to be on bimanual exam
- Perforation made by uterine sound usually occurs in midline posterior uterine wall when there is marked flexion:
  - Remove uterine sound
  - If no bleeding seen, stable BP and pulse, patient pain free and hematocrit stable for next several hours, she may be sent home. Provide alternate contraception
  - If any persistent pain or signs of other organ damage, take or refer immediately for laparoscopic evaluation (extremely rare)
- If IUD perforates acutely, attempt removal by gently pulling on strings
  - If resistance encountered, stop and do pelvic ultrasound and/or send to surgery for immediate laparoscopic IUD removal
- If IUD perforation noted and confirmed by ultrasound at later date, arrange for elective laparoscopic removal

Spotting, frequent or heavy bleeding, hemorrhage, anemia:
- Rule out pregnancy. If pregnant, rule out ectopic pregnancy
- Rule out infection, especially if post-coital bleeding
- Rule out expulsion or partial expulsion of IUD (see below)
- Assess for anemia by lab test; if anemic, provide iron supplement and deal with cause
- Offer NSAIDs every month to reduce bleeding
- Consider replacement with hormonal IUD

Cramping and/or pain:
- Rule out pregnancy, infection, IUD expulsion
- Offer NSAIDs with menses or just before menses every month to reduce cramping
- Consider IUD removal and use of hormonal IUD or another method if problem persists

Expulsion/partial expulsion:
- If expulsion confirmed (IUD seen by patient or clinician), rule out pregnancy
- If expulsion suspected, do ultrasound to determine IUD absence or presence and location. Probe endocervical canal for IUD, remove if present. May replace immediately if patient not pregnant

Strings not felt:
- Check vagina for strings. Assess string length. If normal, reassure and re-instruct patient how to feel for strings
- If strings missing, do pregnancy test and ultrasound to determine if IUD has been expelled. Select next step below according to outcome

Missing strings in non-pregnant patients:
- Twist cytobrush inside cervix to snag strings which may have become snarled in canal
- Examine cervix with uterine sound or visualize canal thru endocervical speculum
- If IUD in endocervix, remove and offer to replace
- If IUD not in cervical canal, after paracervical block, attempt to remove with alligator forceps (some clinicians obtain informed consent after reviewing risks of procedure) or refer for ultrasound to localize prior to attempted removal (provide interim birth control). A 5mm Novak currette and/or intraoperative sonography may be useful in removal of IUDs. In non-pregnant patients, removal may also be done under direct hysteroscopic visualization
- Often can locate IUD with ultrasound. If in place may do nothing. If removal necessary, may remove with ultrasound guidance

Missing strings in pregnant patients:
- Rule out ectopic pregnancy: 5-8% of all failures with the copper IUD are ectopic
- If intrauterine pregnancy, obtain ultrasound to verify IUD in situ

- If IUD is in uterus, advise patient she is at increased risk for preterm labor and spontaneous abortion but reassure her that fetus is not at increased risk for birth defects. May remove IUD at surgery if patient desires elective abortion. Otherwise, plan for removal at delivery
- Reconfirm written consent

Pregnancy with visible strings:
- Visible strings in first trimester: advise removal of IUD to reduce risk of spontaneous abortion and premature labor
- Patient having miscarriage: Remove IUD. Consider antibiotics for 7 days

Infection with IUD use:
- *BV or candidiasis:* treat routinely
- *Trichomoniasis:* treat and reassess IUD candidacy
- *Cervicitis or PID:* Give first dose of antibiotics to achieve adequate serum levels before removing IUD. IUD removal not necessary unless no improvement after antibiotic Rx. Patient may not be candidate for continued IUD use ←
- *Actinomycosis:* Culture of asymptomatic women without an IUD AND of women with an IUD both find that 3-4% are positive for Actinomyces *[Lippes, J. Am J Obstet Gyn-1999; 180-2 65-9].* Often suggested by Pap smear report of "Actinomycosis-like organisms". True upper tract infection with this organism is very serious and requires at least prolonged IV antibiotic therapy with penicillin. However, less than half of women with such Pap smear reports have actinomyces and those that do usually have asymptomatic colonization only. Examine patient for any signs of PID (it can be unilateral). If patient has no clinical evidence of upper tract involvement, 3 major options are available:
  1. Conservative. Annual pap smears only. Advise patient to return as needed or if she develops PID symptoms *or*
  2. Treat with antibiotic penicillin G (500 mg qid p.o. x 1 month) or a tetracycline(tetracycline 500 mg qid p.o. for a month OR doxycycline 100 mg bid x 1 month) and repeat Pap smear *or*
  3. Remove IUD, treat with antibiotic, and repeat Pap smear in 1 month. Reinsert if colonization cleared

REMOVAL

Indications: Expelling IUD, infection, pregnant, expired IUD, complications with IUD, anemia, no longer candidate for IUD, patient request.
Procedure: Grasp the strings close to external os and steadily retract until IUD removed
Complications
- Embedded IUD: Gentle rotation of strings may free IUD. If still stuck, may use alligator forceps removal with or without sonographic guidance (see Missing strings, p. 83). Hysteroscopic removal may be indicated in rare cases. A paracervical block reduces pain from removal of an embedded IUD
- Broken strings: Remove IUD with alligator forceps or Novak curette ←

FERTILITY AFTER USE: Rapid return to baseline fertility

PROGESTERONE IUD (Progestasert® System) (see 2001-2002 Edition)
- No longer marketed for sale in United States

LEVONORGESTREL INTRAUTERINE SYSTEM (Mirena®)

DESCRIPTION: T-shaped intrauterine contraceptive placed within uterine cavity that releases 20 micrograms/day of levonorgestrel from its vertical reservoir. Serum levels of levonorgestrel peak at 25% of the level in POP users taking Ovrette; levels half of those with Norplant. Mirena product information, ordering and reimbursement questions: 1-866-647-3646 (toll free). This IUD has 2 gray strings

EFFECTIVENESS: Effective for up to 10 years *[Speroff-Darney, 2001, page 229]* ◄
Perfect use failure rate in first year: 0.1% (See Table 13.2, p. 38)
Typical use failure rate in first year: 0.1% *[Trussell J. IN Contraceptive Technology, 2004]*
5-year failure rate: 0.7%
• 1-year continuation rate in Finland - 93%; 2 years - 87% *[Bachman-BJOG, 2000]*

MECHANISM: Levonorgestrel causes cervical mucus to become thicker, so sperm can not enter upper reproductive tract and do not reach ovum. Changes in uterotubal fluid also impair sperm migration. Alteration of the endometrium prevents implantation of fertilized ovum. This IUD has some anovulatory effect (5-15% of treatment cycles)

COST: $300-400 (Average wholesale price $395)
• The ARCH Foundation supplies Mirena intrauterine contraceptives to providers caring for economically disadvantaged women whose insurance does not cover Mirena. They ◄ also provide funds for removal to qualifying individuals. Contact your local Berlex representative for information or go to www.archfoundation.com
• Mirena units that are contaminated or must be removed in first 3 months may be replaced free of cost if provider had formal insertion training. Contact Berlex: 1-877-393-9071 ◄ Fax: 704-357-0036

ADVANTAGES
Menstrual:
  • Menorrhagia generally improves (90% with LNg IUS vs. 50% with COCs and 30% with PG inhibitors).
  • Among 44 menorrhagic women receiving Mirena, only 2 were still menorrhagic at 3 ◄ months. In fact, at 9 and 12 months 21 of 44 were amenorrheic *[Monteiro - 2002]*
  • Dysmenorrhea generally improves
  • After 3 to 4 months of menstrual irregularities (mostly spotting), Mirena decreases menstrual blood loss more than 70% (97% reduction in menstrual blood loss in one study) *[Monteiro - 2002]*
  • Amenorrhea develops in approximately 20% of users by 1 year and in 60% by 5 years
  • Decreased surgery (hysterectomies, endometrial ablation, D & C) for menorrhagia, ◄ leiomyomata or adenomeiosis
Sexual/psychological:
  • Convenient: permits spontaneous sexual activity. Requires no action at time of intercourse
  • Reduced fear of pregnancy can make sex more pleasurable
Cancers, tumors and masses: May have protective effect against endometrial cancer
Other:
  • Safe, extremely effective; as effective or more effective than female sterilization
  • May decrease by 60% a woman's risk for PID
  • May be used as the progestin by women on HRT (off-label)
  • *Decreased* risk for ectopic pregnancy
  • May reduce occurrence of endometrial polyps in breast cancer patients taking tamoxifen. Safely of LNg IUS NOT documented in breast Ca patients ◄

DISADVANTAGES
Menstrual: (Removal for any bleeding problem in first year: 7.6%)
  • Number of spotting and bleeding days is significantly higher than normal for first few months ◄ and lower than normal after 3 to 6 months of using levonorgestrel intrauterine system
  • Amenorrhea (a negative if not explained, a positive for some women if explained well in advance) occurs in about 20% of women at one year of use
  • Expulsion: 2.9% in women using Mirena exclusively for contraception; 8.9% to 13.6% ◄ in women using Mirena to control heavy bleeding *[Diaz, 2000] [Monteiro, 2002]*

Sexual/psychological: Same as Copper IUD except when spotting and bleeding may interfere with sexual activity

Other:
- Offers no protection against STIs, except perhaps PID
- May be expelled (median expulsion rate of 4.8% in 19 studies cited in product monograph)
- Persistent unruptured follicles may cause ovarian cysts; most regress spontaneously
- Headaches, acne, mastalgia during first months (very low rates)
- Brief discomfort after insertion or removal

COMPLICATIONS: See 2001 WHO Medical Eligibility Criteria - Appendix: A1 - A8
- PID risk transiently increased after insertion; ovarian cysts
- Allergy to levonorgestrel (rare)
- Perforation of uterus at time of insertion (less than 1 in 1000)

CANDIDATES FOR USE
- Women wanting long-term contraception but wanting to avoid tubal sterilization. While in place, as effective as tubal sterilization
- Can be used in women with heavy menses, cramps or anemia, or DUB who cannot use Copper IUD
- Menopausal women using ERT, with intact uteri, who are unable to tolerate oral progestins are protected against endometrial carcinoma by using a levonorgestrel intrauterine contraceptive *[Raudaskoski, 1995] [Luukkainen, Steroids - 2000]* (off-label)

PRESCRIBING PRECAUTIONS: See WHO Precautions in Appendix: A-1 - A-8 ◀
- May be used by woman with PH of ectopic pregnancy (WHO:1) although packaging says to avoid use in women with risk factors for ectopic pregnancy

INITIATING METHOD: *Each step should be performed slowly and gently*
- *The one-hand insertion technique is different from current Copper IUDs. Training sessions may be set up by calling 1-866-LNG-IUS1.* See Figure 25.3, pages 89-92
- Usually inserted within 7 days of onset of menses to allow hormone levels to be established prior to ovulation
- If no pregnancy exists, it may be possible to insert at other times of cycle
- Insertion tube is 2 mm wider than for copper intrauterine contraceptives; may rarely need to dilate cervix
- A local anesthetic (paracervical block) may be required in some patients, especially ◀ nulliparous patients
- Counsel in advance to expect menstrual cycle changes, including amenorrhea ◀
- Advise NSAIDs for post-insertion discomfort. If pain persists, she must return

INSTRUCTIONS FOR PATIENT: Similar to copper intrauterine contraceptive, p. 84

FOLLOW-UP: Same as Copper IUD

PROBLEM MANAGEMENT: Similar to Copper T 380-A; see p. 85-86

FERTILITY AFTER USE: Immediate return to baseline fertility

Figure 25.3 How to insert Mirena IUS

Preparation for insertion:

- Confirm that the patient understands the method and alternatives and has signed a consent form

- Administer NSAIDS (preferably 1 hour prior to insertion)

- Examine the patient to establish the size and position of the uterus to detect cervicitis or other genital contraindications and to exclude pregnancy.

- **If indicated**, do a vaginal wet mount, obtain cervical cultures, perform a pregnancy test

- Use aseptic technique during insertion. Sterile gloves not needed. Use sterile gloves when learning to insert this IUD. Then can insert using "no-touch technique"

- Cleanse the cervix and vagina with an antiseptic solution

- Administer paracervical block if needed

- Grasp the upper lip of the cervix with a tenaculum and apply gentle traction to align the cervical canal with the uterine cavity and to stabilize cervix

- Carefully sound the uterus to measure its depth and to check the patency of the cervix. If you encounter cervical stenosis, use dilatation, not force, to overcome resistance

- The uterus should sound to a depth of 6 to 9 cm. Insertion of MIRENA into a uterine cavity less than 6.0 cm by sounding may increase the incidence of expulsion, bleeding, pain, perforation and, possibly, pregnancy. (No data on use of Mirena IUS in women with uterus sounding less than 6.0 cm. Mirena insertion may be attempted)

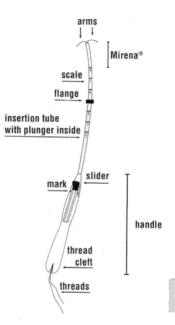

MIRENA® and Inserter

Insertion Procedure:

- Open the sterile package

- Place sterile gloves on your hands or prepare IUS within sterile package

- Pick up the inserter containing MIRENA®

- Carefully release the threads from behind the slider, so that they hang freely

- Make sure that the slider is in the furthest position away from you (positioned at the top of the handle nearest the IUS)

- While looking at the insertion tube, check that the arms of the system are horizontal. If not, align them on a sterile surface or with sterile gloved fingers. This step may be accomplished within sterile package

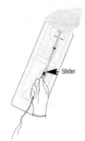

Slider

Checking that the arms of the system are horizontal

- Place the device and the end of the inserter on a sterile surface and pull on both threads to draw the MIRENA® system into the insertion tube (figure a)

- Note that the knobs at the end of the arms now cover the open end of the inserter (figure b)

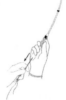

a) MIRENA® system being drawn into the insertion tube

b) The knobs at the ends of the arms

- Fix the threads in the cleft at end of the handle. If too tight they will not come out and then you will pull the IUD out

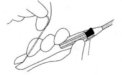

Threads are fixed tightly in the cleft

- Set the flange to the depth measured by the sound This may be accomplished using sterile gloves OR by placing the insertion tube back into the sterile pack and manipulating from the outside. If placed back into sterile pack you do not need an extra sterile surface or sterile gloves

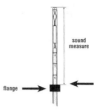

The sound measure

- MIRENA® is now ready to be inserted. Hold the slider firmly in the furthermost position (at the top of the handle). Keep thumb on slider as you insert the inserter. If os is tight and your thumb isn't holding this in place the inserter slides back and the Mirena unloads into the cervix. Grasp the cervix with the tenaculum and apply gentle traction to align the cervical canal with the uterine cavity. Gently insert the inserter into the cervical canal and advance the insertion tube into the uterus until the flange is situated at a distance of about 1.5-2 cm from the external cervical os to give sufficient space for the arms to open. **NOTE: Do not force the inserter**

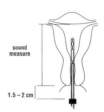

Flange adjusted to sound depth

- While holding the inserter steady, release the arms of MIRENA® by pulling the slider back until the top of the slider reaches the mark (raised horizontal line on the handle). Wait 30 seconds to allow arms to open within the endometrial cavity

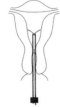

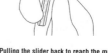

The arms of the MIRENA® being released   **Pulling the slider back to reach the mark**

- Advance the inserter gently into the uterine cavity until the flange touches the cervix. MIRENA® should now be in the fundal position

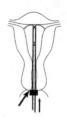

MIRENA® in the fundal position

- Holding the inserter firmly in position release MIRENA® by pulling the slider down all the way. The threads will be released automatically from the cleft

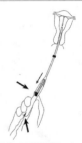

Releasing MIRENA® and withdrawing the inserter

- Remove the inserter from the uterus. Cut the threads to leave about 3-5 cm visible outside the cervix. Be sure not to displace the Mirena IUS if cutting the strings with dull scissors. Give cut strings to patient ◄— to feel and to keep

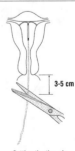

3-5 cm

Cutting the threads

PILLS – DAILY "THE PILL" COMBINED PILLS

DESCRIPTION: Each hormonally active pill in combined pills contains an estrogen and a progestin. Ethinyl estradiol (EE) is the most commonly used estrogen; it is in most 50 µg pills and all of the sub-50 µg formulations. Mestranol, which must be metabolized to EE to become biologically active, is found in two 50 µg formulations (rarely prescribed). At least 7 progestins are used in the different pill formulations. All packs have 21 active combined pills, with or without 7 additional pills (usually placebo pills). **Monophasic formulations contain active pills with the same amount of hormones in each tablet.** Multiphasic formulations contain active pills with varying amounts of progestin and/or estrogen in the active pills of the cycle. One formulation (Mircette) has the traditional 21 days of active pills followed by 2 days of placebo pills and 5 days of pills with 10 µg EE alone. Another, Seasonale, has 84 consecutive hormonal pills

Yasmin, with drospirenone, has antimineralocorticoid properties. While formally approved for none of these conditions, it may be useful for women with PMDD - premenstrual dysphoric disorder, PMS, acne, hirsutism and PCOS *[Krattenmacher-2000]*. Drospirenone may increase postassium and women on certain medications should have a blood test to check their potassium level after the first month of taking Yasmin (see bottom of Fig. 26.2 on p. 106)

EFFECTIVENESS

Perfect use failure rate in first year: 0.3% (of every 1,000 women who take pills for 1 year, 3 will become pregnant in the year of use) (See Table 13.2, p. 38)
Typical use failure rate in first year: 8% *[Trussell J IN Contraceptive Technology, 2004]*

MECHANISM: Suppresses ovulation (90% to 95% of time). Also causes thickening of cervical mucus, which blocks sperm penetration and entry into the upper reproductive tract. Thin, asynchronous endometrium inhibits implantation. Tubal and endometrial motility slowed.

COST

- Cost of one cycle: from a few dollars to more than $50. Most pharmacies charge $20-42/cycle
- Costs differ from region to region, and pills with 50 mcg of estrogen often cost more.
- Generic brands are generally less expensive. They are not required to have clinical testing; they must only prove blood level equivalency (80–125% of parent compound's blood levels). There is NO evidence that generics are less effective than brand name products
- canadiandrugstore.com will provide COCs at 1/2 to 1/3 the cost.
- Most major insurance companies cover pills

ADVANTAGES
Menstrual:
- Decreased blood loss and decreased anemia may decrease menstrual cramps/pain, and more predictable menses
- Eliminates ovulation pain (Mittelschmerz)
- Can be used to manipulate timing and frequency of menses (see Choice of COC, p. 104 & 108)
- Reduces risk of internal hemorrhage from ovulation (especially important in women with bleeding diatheses or women using anticoagulants)
- Regulates menses in women with anovulation/PCOS

Sexual/psychological:
- No disruption at time of intercourse; more spontaneous activity
- Enhanced sexual enjoyment due to diminished risk of pregnancy

Cancers/tumors/masses:
- A case control study of US women found that even low-estrogen and low progestin OCs ◄ offer the same 50% reduction in ovarian cancer risk as higher-dose formulations *[Ness-2000]*. COC users for 5 years have 50% reduction in risk; users for 10 years have 80% reduction. Protection extends for 30 years beyond last pill use; Significant reduction in risk also seen in some high risk women carrying BRCA mutations
- Decreased risk for **endometrial cancer** *[Grimes-2001]* (clearly demonstrated for 30 μg and higher dose pills)
  - COC users for 1 year have 20% reduction in risk; users for 4 years have 60% reduction
  - Protection extends for 30 years beyond last pill use *[Ness, AmJEpidemiol-2000]*
  - Particularly important for PCOS women, obese women, and perimenopausal women
- Decreased risk of death from **colorectal cancer** seen in current COC users and in women who used COCs within the last 10 years *[Berel-1999]*
- Decreased risk of corpus luteum cysts and hemorrhagic corpus luteum cysts
- *Breast masses:* 25% reduction in all **benign breast disease** (including fibroadenomas)

DO BIRTH CONTROL PILLS CAUSE BREAST CANCER?

- ► After more than 50 studies, most experts believe *that pills have little, if any, effect on the risk of developing breast cancer.*
- ► The Women's Care Study of 4575 women with breast cancer and 4682 controls found no increased risk for breast cancer (RR: 1.0) among women currently using pills and a decreased risk of breast cancer (RR: 0.9) for those women who had previously used pills. Use of pills by women with a family history of breast cancer was not associated with an increased risks of breast cancer, nor was the initiation of pill use at a young age *[Marchbanks - 2002]*
- However, several studies have shown that current users of pills are slightly more likely to be *diagnosed* with breast cancer (Relative Risk: 1.2). *[Collaborative Group; Lancet 1996]*
- Two factors may explain the increased risk of breast cancer being diagnosed in women currently taking pills: 1) *detection bias* (more breast exams and more mammography) or 2) *promotion* of an already present nidus of cancer cells
- Ten years after discontinuing pills, women who have taken pills are at no increased risk for having breast cancer diagnosed. *[Collaborative Group; Lancet 1996]*
- Breast cancers diagnosed in women currently on pills or women who have taken pills in the past are more likely to be localized *(less likely to be metastatic)*. *[Collaborative Group; Lancet 1996]*
- By the age of 55, the risk of having had breast cancer diagnosed is the same for women who have used pills and those who have not
- The conclusion of the largest collaborative study of the risk for breast cancer is that women with a strong family Hx of breast cancer do not further increase their risk for breast cancer risk by taking pills. *[Collaborative Group; Lancet 1996]* This was also the conclusion of the Nurses Health Study *[Lipnick - 1986] [Colditz - 1996]* and the Cancer and Steroid Hormone (CASH) study. *[Murray - 1989] [The Centers for Disease Control Cancer and Steroid Hormone Study - 1983]*
- While there are still unanswered questions about pills and breast cancer, today, four decades after their arrival on the contraceptive scene, the overall conclusion is that pills do not cause breast cancer. *"Many years after stopping oral contraceptive use, the main effect may be protection against metastatic disease."* *[Speroff and Darney - 2001]* *[Collaborative Group; Lancet 1996]*

Other:

- Reduces risk of hospitalization with diagnosis of PID
- Reduces risk of ectopic pregnancy
- Treatment for acne, hirsutism and other androgen excess states
- Reduced vasomotor symptoms and effective contraception in perimenopausal women ◄━
- Increased bone mineral density when pills with 35 micrograms of estrogen used by women in their 40s; have been found to reduce postmenopausal hip fractures *[Michaelsson-1998; Lancet, 353:1481-1484]*. 20 mcg pills likely to have similar benefit

DISADVANTAGES

Menstrual:

- Spotting, particularly during first few cycles and with inconsistent use
- Scant or missed menses possible, not clinically significant but can cause worry
- Post-pill amenorrhea (lasts up to 6 months). Uncommon and usually in women with history of irregular periods prior to taking pills

Sexual/psychological:

- Decreased libido and anorgasms are possible, but unusual. COCs blunt midcycle ◄━ testosterone peak
- Mood changes, depression, anxiety, irritability, fatigue may develop while on COCs
  - Rule out other causes before implicating COCs
- Daily pill taking may be stressful (especially if privacy is an issue)

Cancers/tumors/masses:

- **Breast cancer: see comprehensive answer in box on previous page**
- **Cervical cancer:**
  - No consistent increased risk seen for squamous cell cervical carcinoma (85% of all cervical cancer) after controlling for confounding variables, such as number of sex partners
  - Risk of a relatively uncommon type of cervical cancer, adenocarcinoma, is increased 60%, but no extra screening required other than recommended Pap screening ◄━
- **Hepatocellular adenoma:** risk increased among COC users (only ≥ 50 μg formulations). Risk of hepatic carcinoma not increased, even in populations with high prevalence of hepatitis B

Other:

- No protection against STIs, including HIV. Must use safe sex practices, including condoms
- Shedding of HIV may be slightly increased ◄━
- Nausea or vomiting, especially in first few cycles
- Breast tenderness or pain, especially in first few cycles; breast enlargement
- Headaches: may increase in frequency and/or intensity
- Increased varicosities, chloasma, capillary spiders (higher estrogen formulations)
- Daily dosing is difficult for some women who cannot remember to take a pill daily
- Weight gain (including significant sustained weight gain in rare women), but average weight gain no different among COC users than placebo users (see NOTE below)
- See COMPLICATIONS section below

NOTE: Medical problems and symptom complaints are frequently attributed by patients and providers to COC use. While some women may be particularly sensitive to sex steroids, a recent placebo-controlled study found that the incidence of all of the frequently mentioned hormone-related side effects was not significantly different in the COC group than it was in the placebo group *[Redmond, 1999]* For example, headaches occurred in 18.4% of women on Ortho Tricyclen and in 20.5% of women in the placebo group. Nausea occurred in 12.7% of women on Ortho Tricyclen and in 9.0 % of women on placebo pills. Weight gain occurred in 2.2% of women on Ortho Tricyclen and in 2.1 % of women on placebo pills

COMPLICATIONS

- *Venous thromboembolism (VTE)*
  - The risk of VTE with COC use is less than with pregnancy:

No COC use	4-8/100,000 women per year
COC use	10-30/100,000 women per year
Pregnancy	60/100,000 women per year

  - DVT risk is associated with the dose of estrogen; the risk of VTE in 50 μg pills is greater than in 20-35 μg pills. The type of progestin may *slightly* influence DVT risk; If true, this risk is still only one-half of the VTE associated with pregnancy.. The current labeling for desogestrel pills states that "several epidemiologic studies indicate that third generation oral contraceptives, including those containing desogestrel, are associated with a higher risk of venous thromboembolism than certain second generations OCs. In general, these studies indicate an approximate 2-fold increased risk, which corresponds to an additional 1-2 cases of venous thromboembolism per 10,000 women-years of use. However, data from additional studies have not shown this 2-fold increase in risk." Neither the U.S. Food & Drug Administration (FDA) nor the American College of Obstetricians (ACOG) recommends switching current users of desogestrel containing pills to other products. Underlying blood dyscrasias such as Factor V_{Leiden} mutation and Protein S or C abnormalities increase risk of VTE significantly. However, in the absence of strong family history (see boxed message on p. 96), routine screening is not necessary. Concern about increased risk in Yasmin ◄── users for DVT may be premature; more studies are needed

- *Myocardial infarction (MI) and stroke*
  - There is no increased risk of MI or stroke for young women who are using low-dose COCs who do not smoke, do not have hypertension and do not have migraine headaches with neurological findings
  - Women at risk:
    - Smokers over 35 shouldn't use COCs; all smokers should be encouraged to stop smoking. Smokers over 35 have MI rate of 396 per million COC users per year vs. 88 per million non-COC users per year
    - Women with hypertension, diabetes, hyperlipidemia or obesity
    - Women with migraine headaches, new onset headaches (only stroke risk increases)
- *Hypertension:* 1% of users develop hypertension which (usually) is reversible within 1-3 months of discontinuing COCs. Most users have a very small increase in blood pressure

---

ELEVATED BLOOD PRESSURE: A TEACHABLE MOMENT

Your very quick advice each time you find an elevated blood pressure might include several messages.

1. If you smoke, stop smoking. It is by far the most important step you can take
2. Exercise regularly. Moderate exercise for 20-30 minutes each day
3. If overweight, lose weight. Reduce fat in your diet
4. Use salt in moderation
5. If you are on antihypertensive medications, take them regularly!
6. Work on reducing stress in your life (may be difficult and may take time)

- *Neoplasia:* COC users using early high dose pills are at higher risk of developing ← adenocarcinoma (rare) of the cervix and hepatic adenomas (rare). See boxed message on p. 94 for an answer to the question: Do birth control pills cause breast cancer?
- *Cholelithiasis/cholecystitis:* higher dose formulations were associated with doubling the risk of symptomatic gallbladder disease
  • Sub-50 mcg formulations may be neutral or have a slightly increased risk
  • Use COCs with caution in women with known gallstones
- *Visual changes:* Rare cases of retinal thrombosis. Contact lens users may have dry eye. May need to recommend eye drops or need to switch methods

CANDIDATES FOR USE

- Most healthy reproductive aged women are candidates for COCs; encourage use of ← condoms if at risk for STIs
- For healthy women, the use of COCs is often decided on the basis of a balance of perceived benefits and side effects. Careful counseling can help patient recognize all the health benefits COCs offer and help motivate her to daily COC use
- Women with conditions listed under prescribing precautions may occasionally be candidates for COC use if the benefits outweigh the risk as discussed in the MEDICAL ELIGIBILITY CHECKLIST section (see p. 100 & Appendix A-1–A-8). However, non-hormonal methods or hormonal methods that do not contain estrogen are generally more appropriate. In addition to medical precautions, real world situations such as the need for privacy, affordable access to COCs, and the requirement for daily administration need to be considered when evaluating a woman for COC use

Adolescents

- May be excellent candidates for contraceptive benefits if patient is able to take a pill each day.
- Many of the non-contraceptive effects of OCs are particularly important for adolescent women – e.g. decreased dysmenorrhea (the most common cause of lost days of school and work among women under 25), and decreased acne, hirsutism, or hypoestrogenism due to eating disorders, excessive exercise, stress, etc.
- Failure rates are higher in teens using COCs. Help teens integrate pill taking into daily rituals (tooth brushing, beeper, watch alarm, application of makeup, putting on earrings).
← Ask teenager how she will create a way to be successful. Ask if parents are aware that she ← is using contraception and if they are supportive. Consider continuous COC use. See p. 99
- If at risk for STIs, encourage teens to also use condoms
- Always discuss and offer advance prescription/provision of Plan B emergency contraceptive pills

SPECIAL CONSIDERATIONS FOR USE

- Women with medical conditions that improve with COCs may find COCs a particularly attractive contraceptive option. This includes women with endometriosis, migraine, iron deficiency anemia, acne, hirsutism, polycystic ovarian syndrome (PCOS), ovarian or endometrial cancer risk factors, eating disorders or activity patterns that increase risk of osteoporosis. Consider continuous COC use with Seasonale or other monophasic pill. ← See p. 99
- Women whose reproductive health would be improved by ovulation suppression or decreased menstrual blood loss should also consider COCs. This includes women who suffer menorrhea or dysmenorrhea, some anticoagulated women (COCs decrease risk of internal hemorrhage with ovulation and menorrhagia) and women using seizure medication (decrease menorrhagia). Certain anti-seizure medications may lower COC effectiveness and require higher dose formulation

- Women whose quality of life would be improved by reducing frequency of or eliminating menses with continuous COC use: See next page

PRESCRIBING PRECAUTIONS

See WHO Eligibility Criteria Appendix A1 - A8

- Thrombophlebitis, thromboembolic disease or history of deep venous thrombosis or pulmonary embolism (unless anticoagulated)
- Family history of close family members with unexplained VTE at an early age (eg Factor V_{Leiden} mutation)

The questions to ask are as follows:

- Has a close family member (parents, siblings, grandparents, uncles, aunts) ever had multiple, unexplained blood clots in the legs or lungs?
- Has a close family member ever been hospitalized for blood clots in the legs or lungs? If so, did this person take a blood thinner? (If not, the likelihood is that the family member may have had a nonsignificant condition such as superficial phlebitis or varicose veins)
- What were the circumstances in which the blood clot took place? (eg. cancer, airline travel, surgery, obesity, immobility, postpartum, etc.)? *[Grimes - 1999]*

"If the family history screening is positive - one or more close family members with a definite strong VTE history (young first - or second - degree relatives with spontaneous VTE) clinician might consider further laboratory screening for genetic conditions. Another alternative is to suggest progestin-only OCs or another non-estrogen-containing birth control method." *[Grimes - 1999]*

- Cerebral vascular disease or coronary artery disease
- Current breast cancer (WHO: 4)
- Past breast cancer and no evidence of current disease for 5 years (WHO: 3)
- Endometrial carcinoma or other estrogen dependent neoplasia (excluding endometriosis and leiomyoma) WHO rates endometrial cancer a "1" for COCs ◄—
- Unexplained vaginal bleeding suspicious for serious condition (before evaluation) (WHO: 2)
- Cholestatic jaundice of pregnancy or jaundice with prior pill use
- Hepatic adenoma or carcinoma or significant hepatic dysfunction
- Smoking after age 35. WHO defines heavy smoking as $\geq$ 15 cigarettes/day (see p. A3) ◄—
- Complicated or prolonged diabetes, systemic lupus erythematosus (if vascular changes)
- Severe migraine with aura or other neurologic symptoms
- Breastfeeding women until 4 months postpartum ◄—
- Hypersensitivity to any components of pills
- Daily use of a broadspectrum antibiotic such as ampicillin/doxycycline. Although WHO ◄— (see p. A8) states that women using antibiotics other than grisiofulvin or rifampicin may use COCs (WHO:1), patients are exposed to conflicting information and many clinicians explain the differing opinons and let patient decide for herself. These are not convincing data that broad specrum antibiotics increase the failure of COCs
- Hypertension with vascular disease $\dfrac{140\text{-}159}{90\text{-}99} = 3$ (WHO) $\dfrac{\geq 160}{\geq 100} = 4$ (WHO) ◄—

CONTINUOUS USE OF COMBINED ORAL CONTRACEPTIVE PILLS (COCS) MAY MEAN:

A. Manipulation of a cycle to delay one period for a trip, honeymoon, or athletic event
B. Use of active hormonal pills (no hormone-free) for 2, 3 or 4 packages (42, 63, 84 consecutive days) followed by 2 to 7 hormone-free days. Seasonale is a COC designed to produce 4 cycles per year. This regimen will be the only approved product for extended-cycle regimen use. It provides COCs for 84 consecutive days followed by 7 hormone-free days. The pills used for Seasonale ARE THE SAME 30 mcg EE pills with levonorgestrel as Nordette, Lo-Ovral, Levlen, Levora. Pills other than Seasonale may be used to accomplish this same end. There is nothing sacred about the 7-day hormone free interval. The hormone-free interval may be less than 7 days (from 0 to 6 days), but should not exceed 7 days
C. Continuous daily COCs until spotting starts. Then a 3 to 7-day break from hormones
D. Use of a monophasic pill indefinitely. BTB can occur at any time with this regimen. Eventually she develops an atrophic endometrium and breakthrough bleeding decreases

Cyclic symptoms that may improve if a woman uses pills continuously include:
Symptoms usually occurring at the time of menses:
• Lower abdominal, back or leg pain or cramping. Pain from endometriosis
• Bleeding, including menorrhagia
• Irritability or depression. Decreased libido
• Headaches including both cyclic migraine and other cyclic headaches
• Nausea, dizziness, vomiting or diarrhea
• Cyclic yeast or other infections or cyclic nosebleeds
• Cyclic seizures or recurrences of asthma at the time of menses
• Changes in insulin requirements

Symptoms usually during at midcycle:
• Secretions associated with high estradiol levels or spotting due to fall in estradiol
• Nausea
• Sharp or dull pain (that precedes ovulation and is caused by high midcycle PG levels)

Symptoms usually occurring just prior to menses:
• Slight to more dramatic weight gain, bloating, swollen eyes or ankles
• Breast fullness or tenderness
• Anxiety, irritability or depression, headaches or nausea
• Acne, spotting, discharge, breast fullness or tenderness
• Pain or cramping or constipation

Most important advantages & disadvantages of taking COCs continuously:
Advantages:
• May be more effective as a contraceptive
• Easier to remember (do the same thing every day)
• Easier for people with hectic lives (e.g. residents and medical students)
• Women wanting to avoid bleeding for an athletic event, special trip or any other reason
• No bleeding each month
• Undesirable cyclic symptoms may be improved
• May reduce symptoms associated with more frequent cycles

Disadvantages:
• More expensive and the extra packs of pills required may not be covered by insurance
• Spotting and the absence of regular menses; considered unnatural by some women

MEDICAL ELIGIBILITY CHECKLIST: Ask client the questions below. If she answers NO to ALL of the questions and has no other contraindications, then she can use low-dose COCs if she wants. If she answers YES to a question below, follow the instructions

1. Do you think you are pregnant?

☐ No ☐ Yes Assess if pregnant. If she might be pregnant, give her condoms or spermicide to use until reasonably certain that she is not pregnant. Then she can start COCs. If unprotected sex within past 5 days, consider emergency contraception if she is not pregnant

2. Do you smoke cigarettes and are you age 35 or older?

☐ No ☐ Yes Urge her to stop smoking. If she is 35 or older and she will not stop smoking, do not provide COCs. Help her choose a method without estrogen

3. Do you have high blood pressure? (see Appendix, p. A2)

☐ No ☐ Yes *If BP below 140/90*, OK to give COCs if no other comorbidities exist even if taking antihypertensive drugs. *If BP is elevated*, see Appendix, p. A-3. Consider POPs

4. Are you breast-feeding your baby?

☐ No ☐ Yes *No controversy*: Provide the COCs she will use when she stops nursing. Also provide interval contraceptive she may use while nursing her baby. *Some controversy*: Provide COCs and counsel to start when she adds nutrition from other sources (formula or solid foods). Provide interval method, give her ECPs and condom. *Controversial, (but supported by clinical studies)*: may start COCs after lactation well established. POPs and other progestin-only methods preferable to COCs as they suppress milk production less

5. Do you have serious medical problems such as a heart disease, severe chest pain, blood clots, high blood pressure or diabetes? Have you ever had such problems?

☐ No ☐ Yes Do not provide COCs if she reports heart attack or heart disease due to blocked arteries, stroke, blood clots (except superficial clots), severe chest pain with unusual shortness of breath, diabetes for more than 20 years, or damage to vision, kidneys, or nervous system caused by diabetes. Help her choose a method without estrogen. Consider POPs, ◀— LNg IUD, Copper T 380 A, Implanon, barriers, DMPA

6. Do you have or have you ever had breast cancer? (see p. A4)

☐ No ☐ Yes Do not provide COCs if current or less than 5 years ago. Help her ◀— choose a method without hormones

7. Do you often get bad headaches with blurred vision, nausea or dizziness?

☐ No ☐ Yes If she gets migraine headaches with blurred vision, temporary loss of vision, sees flashing lights or zigzag lines, or trouble speaking or moving, or has other neurologic symptoms, do not provide COCs. If she has only menstrual migraines without abnormal neurologic findings, consider COC use (see choice of COC use, p. 106). Help her choose a method without estrogen. Consider POPs, LNg IUD, Copper T 380 A, Implanon, barriers ◀—

8. Are you taking medicine for seizures? Are you taking rifampin, griseofulvin or St. John's Wort? ◀—

☐ No ☐ Yes If she has no breakthrough bleeding, she can continue using only the pill. If she is using St. John's Wort, rifampin or griseofulvin, guide her to DMPA or a non-hormonal method or strongly encourage condom use as backup contraceptive. If she is taking topiramate (Topomax) phenytoin, carbamazepine, barbiturates, or primidone for seizures, provide condoms as backup contraceptive. Consider raising dose of COCs to 50 µg EE pills, or help her choose another effective method if she is on long-term treatment. She may be able to use 35-µg pills.

Some have suggested using condoms as a backup. Use of valproic acid does NOT lower the effectiveness of COCs. See discussion p. 103

9. Do you have vaginal bleeding that is unusual for you? (see Appendix, p. A3)

☐ No ☐ Yes If she is not likely to be pregnant but has unexplained vaginal bleeding that suggests an underlying medical condition, evaluate condition before initiating pills. Treat as appropriate or refer. Reassess COC use based on findings

10. Do you have jaundice, cirrhosis of the liver, an acute liver infection or tumor? (Are her eyes or skin unusually yellow?) (see p. A5)

☐ No ☐ Yes If she has serious active liver disease (jaundice, painful or enlarged liver, active viral hepatitis, liver tumor), do not provide COCs. Refer for care as appropriate. Help her choose a method without hormones

11. Do you have gallbladder disease? Ever had jaundice while taking COCs or during pregnancy?

☐ No ☐ Yes If she has acute gallbladder disease now or takes medicine for gallbladder disease, or if she has had jaundice while using COCs or during pregnancy, do not provide COCs. Consider a method without estrogen. Women with known asymptomatic cholelithiasis may use COCs with caution

12. Are you planning surgery with a recovery period that will keep you from walking for a week or more? Have you had a baby in the past 21 days?

☐ No ☐ Yes Help her choose a method without estrogen. If planning surgery or just had a baby, provide COCs for delayed initiation and another interim method

13. Have you ever gotten pregnant on the pill?

☐ No ☐ Yes Ask about pill-taking habits. Consider longer dosing hormonal methods or shortening or eliminating the pill-free interval while using COCs

INITIATING METHOD (see INSTRUCTIONS FOR PATIENT, p. 103)

- In asymptomatic women, **a pelvic examination is not necessary to start pills** *[Stewart-2001]*
- *Counseling is critical in helping women successfully use the pill*
  - Patients who are counseled well about how to use pills and what side effects may develop are usually better prepared and may be more likely to continue use
- *Timing of initiation* (see Table 26.2, p. 105)
  - **First day of next menstrual period start is generally preferred because no routine backup method is needed**
  - If using Sunday start, recommend back-up method x 7 days. Sunday start leads to ◄— no periods on weekends
  - "Same day start" (starting the day of the counseling clinic visit) is quite feasible to help women (especially teens) adapt to COCs but provide 7 day backup
- *Choice of pill*
  - The pill that will work best for the woman is the one that she will take regularly
  - For special situations, some formulations offer advantages over others (see CHOOSING COCs FOR WOMEN IN SPECIAL SITUATIONS, next page)

- In general, use the lowest dose of hormones that will provide pregnancy protection, deliver the non-contraceptive benefits that are important to the woman, and minimize her side effects
- Monophasic formulations are preferable if women are interested in controlling cycle lengths or timing by eliminating any or all pill-free intervals for medical indications or personal preference (see Choosing COCs, Figure 26.2 p. 106)
- Triphasic formulations may be preferable to use to reduce some side effects (such as premenstrual breakthrough bleeding) when it is not desirable to increase hormone levels throughout the entire cycle or when it is desirable to reduce total cycle progestin levels (e.g. acne treatment). There is no definite research indicating the superiority of triphasic pills for women with BTB
- *Choice of pattern of COC use*
  - 28-day cycling: Most common use pattern. Women have monthly withdrawal bleeding during placebo pills
  - *"First day start" each cycle:* Women can start each new pack of pills on first day of menses each cycle
  - *"Bicycling" or "tricycling":* Women skip placebo pills for either 1 or 2 packs and then use the placebo pills and have withdrawal bleeding every 7 weeks (end of 2nd pack) or 10 weeks (end of 3rd pack). **Use monophasic pills**
  - You may prescribe 4 packs of low dose monophasic pills omitting the placebo pills. The new pill, *Seasonale,* will be packaged to provide pills in this manner: 84 active pills followed by 7 days of inactive pills, resulting in 4 withdrawal bleeds/year ◄—
  - *"Continuous use":* Women take only active pills and have no withdrawal bleeding. Often women must transition through bicycling or tricycling to achieve amenorrhea. Must use monophasic pills. Need to counsel regarding BTB and spotting
  - *NOTE: the last three options may be particularly good for:*
    - Women with menstrually-related problems (menorrhagia, anemia, dysmenorrhea, menstrual mood changes, menstrual irregularity, endometriosis, menstrual migraine, PMS, PMDD)
    - Women on medications that reduce COC effectiveness (e.g. anticonvulsants, St. John's Wort)
    - Women who have conceived while on COCs or who forget to take them regularly
    - Women who are ambulatory but disabled (not wheelchair bound) ◄—
    - Women who want to control their cycles for their own convenience

CHOOSING COCs FOR WOMEN IN SPECIAL SITUATIONS

- *Diabetes and glucose intolerance:* low-dose pills with lower progestin content and low androgenicity to reduce insulin resistance and cardiovascular risks
- *Endometriosis:* relatively strong progestin content helpful to create pseudo-pregnancy state. Seasonale and other pills taken continuously are most effective in reducing symptoms. Continuous use (no break) of Lunelle, ring or patch are also probably effective ◄—
- *Functional ovarian cysts:* higher dose COCs more effective. If using 50 µg formulations, select one with EE for maximum effectiveness. Low dose pills have less or no protective effect vs. cysts
- *Androgen excess states:* all COCs are helpful but pills with higher estrogen/progestin ratios are preferable to reduce free testosterone and inhibit 5 alpha-reductase activity
- *Breastfeeding women:* progestin-only methods preferable to COCs in breastfeeding ◄— women. COCs may be considered when baby's diet supplemented by other sources of nutrition or after lactation well established (if patient prefers COCs)

- *Hypercholesterolemia:* Selection of pill depends on type of dyslipidemia:
  - Elevated LDL or low HDL: consider estrogenic pill (high estrogen/progestin ratio) with low androgenicity
  - Elevated triglycerides: Some clinicians recommend not prescribing COCs if triglycerides > 350 mg/dL because COCs increase triglycerides by approximately 30% and risk of pancreatitis increased (norgestimate may increase triglycerides less) ◄
- *Hepatic enzyme-inducing agents (e.g. anticonvulsants except valproic acid and St. John's Wort):* Options:
  - Prescribe high-dose COC (containing 50 µg EE)
  - Prescribe 30-35 µg pill with reduced pill-free interval (first-day start, bicycling with first day start, or continuous use)
  - Prescribe 35 µg pill and use backup for 3 cycles. If no breakthrough bleeding by third cycle, discontinue backup method. If she has breakthrough bleeding, increase hormone levels or continue use of backup method (least reliable technique)
- *Antibiotic use:* Concern that without intestinal flora to unconjugate the hormonal compounds produced by first hepatic processing, subsequent reabsorption of estrogen and progestin would not be possible. However, recent research suggests <u>no</u> significant difference in circulating serum levels of hormones when women used broad-spectrum antibiotics. Class OC labeling warns about potential antibiotic interaction. If patient has other risk factor (vomiting, diarrhea, forgetfulness) or prefers, suggest back-up method for duration of antibiotic use. Griseofulvin and rifampin <u>do</u> decrease pill effectiveness ◄
- *Obese patient:* Concern for thrombosis with higher dose estrogen; one retrospective study found ◄ pregnancy rates increased greatly, especially if 20 mcg formulations given to women over 154 pounds

INSTRUCTIONS FOR PATIENT: Periodic "breaks" from pills are NOT recommended!

- Key to successful pill use is a well-informed patient. Provide new-start patients with:
  - Clear instructions on pill initiation, preferably written and in her primary language. If reasonably certain that she is not pregnant use Quick Start technique *[Westoff - 2002]*. ◄ Have her take the first hormonally active pill immediately and use all pills. This will delay onset of next period. This will delay onset of next period. This will not increase the number of days of menstrual bleeding nor the number of days of spotting. The 3 month continuation rate among Quick Start women was markedly better than women starting pills at later times
  - Help her plan where to store pills, how to remember to take them and where to obtain refills
  - Explanation about possible transitional side effects (spotting, breast tenderness, headaches, etc.) and encouragement to call or return should any become troublesome (see PROBLEM MANAGEMENT). Also highlight noncontraceptive benefits
    - Warning about serious complications (see ACHES, Figure 26.1 & p. A-23)
- Backup method: ensure patient has and knows how to use method if she needs to use one for interim protection, back-up, or as an alternate method if she ever discontinues COC use. Provide ECPs ◄
- Have patient return in 3 months for BP check and follow-up of any complaints. Subsequently, only annual routine gynecologic exams are offered to low-risk patients
- Provide ECPs to use if she has missed pills

FOLLOW-UP CHECKLIST AT EACH RETURN VISIT:

- **Do you take your pills every single day? (see PROBLEM MANAGEMENT)**
- Are you having any symptoms of pregnancy?
- Are you having any changes in your periods? (see Figure 26.3 on page 107)
- Are you having any breast tenderness, upset stomach, increased acne, mood changes, changes in your sex life, weight changes, headaches or other health problems?

- What medications are you taking?
- How much do you smoke?
- Are you having any of the ACHES problems? (See appendix, p. A-23)
- Do you plan to have children? OR Do you plan to have more children?
- Do you have any other problems you think might be related to taking pills?

Figure 26.1 PILL WARNING SIGNALS (ACHES) see also Appendix (A-23)

ACHES: A way to remember pill danger signals
A   Abdominal pain? Yellow skin or eyes?
C   Chest pain?
H   Headaches that are severe?
E   Eye problems: blurred vision or loss of vision?
S   Severe leg pain or swelling (in the calf or thigh)?
If you are experiencing depression, speak to your clinician   ◀

PROBLEM MANAGEMENT

Nausea/vomiting: **Rule out pregnancy, reassure that nausea usually improves**

- Suggest taking pills at night (evening meal or bedtime) to allow patient to sleep through high serum levels of hormones. Suggest taking pills with morning meal if experiencing bothersome nausea during the night
- If patient vomits within one hour of taking pill, suggest antiemetic prior to taking replacement pill. Use backup method for 7 days ◀
- Abdominal pain problems possibly related to COCs: thombosis of major intra-abdominal vessels, gallstones, pancreatitis, liver adenoma, Crohn's disease or porphyria

Spotting and/or breakthrough bleeding: (see Figure 26.3, p. 107)

Missed one pill: **Instruct patient to take missed pill ASAP and take next pill as usual**

- Offer emergency contraceptive pills (ECPs), especially if missed pill is at beginning of pack.
- WHO (2002) She does NOT need any additional contraception (including ECPs)

Missed two pills:

- Instruct patient to take one of the forgotten pills every 12 hours until she gets caught up, then continue rest of pack. Suggest long-acting antiemetic one hour before second pill if drowsiness is not a problem. Backup contraception recommended for 7 days
- Alternatively, offer ECPs, especially if patient is early in cycle and restart COCs next day

Missed more than two pills: **Actually, provide ECPs in advance** ◀

- If patient declines ECPs, instruct patient to skip missed pills and complete rest of pills in pack, but to use barrier method with each act of intercourse until her next menses. Advise patient that pills may not provide protection, but will help control her cycle

If patient uses ECPs: **Advise patient to skip the missed COCs in her pack**

- Instruct patient to resume taking pills in pack the next day after she finishes ECPs

Missed menses on COCs:

- Offer pregnancy test, especially if she missed any pills in last cycle or if she has any symptoms of pregnancy
- Offer emergency contraception if any recent unprotected intercourse
- Advise patient that there are no adverse clinical impacts of amenorrhea from COCs
- If patient prefers monthly menses, consider switching to formulation with higher estrogen or lower progestin
- Otherwise, have her continue her COCs on usual schedule

New onset or significant worsening of headaches on COCs: (see Figure 26.4, p. 108)

Hot flashes on placebo-pill week:
- Suggest starting on first day of menses or continuous use of monophasic pills OR
- Offer low-dose of transdermal or oral estrogen during placebo-pill week

MAKING THE TRANSITION FROM COCs TO HRT: (See Figure 26.5, p. 109)

FERTILITY AFTER USE

- Rapid return to fertility: Average delay in ovulation 1-2 weeks. Rarely, post-pill amenorrhea may persist for up to 6 months. Post-pill amenorrhea is usually in women with history of very irregular menses prior to initiating pills
- Women should initiate another method immediately after discontinuing COCs
- Women should be advised that their pattern of menses prior to starting pills (frequency, duration, flow, dysmenorrhea) tends to return once they stop COCs

Table 26.2 Starting Combined Oral Contraceptives*

CONDITION BEFORE STARTING	WHEN TO START COCs?
Starting (restarting) COCs in menstruating women	• Immediately, if pregnancy excluded start with first pill in package or with pill appropriate for her cycle day** "QUICK START" [Westoff - 2002] ◄ • First day of next menses (preferable) • Within 5 days after start of her menstrual bleeding. No backup contraception is needed • First Sunday after next menses begins**
Starting (restarting) in amenorrheic women	Anytime it is reasonably certain that she is not pregnant; abstain from sex or use backup method for next 7 days
Postpartum and breast-feeding	If still breastfeeding & less than 6 months PP, wait at least until the baby is receiving significant nutritional supplement If more than 6 months PP & amenorrheic, start COCs as advised for other amenorrheic woman
Postpartum and not breast-feeding (after pregnancy of 24 or more weeks)	• Wait 3 weeks after delivery to allow hypercoagulable state of pregnancy to abate
After 1st or 2nd trimester (≤ 24 weeks) pregnancy loss or termination	• Immediately - QUICK START [Westoff - 2002]
Switching from another hormonal method	• Start COCs immediately (QUICK START) if she has been using hormonal method correctly and consistently , or if it is reasonably certain she is not pregnant. No need to wait until next period. No additional contraceptive needed • If previous method was an injectable start COCs at the time repeat injection would have been given
Switching from a non-hormonal non-hormonal method (other than IUD)	• Can start COCs within 5 days after start of her menstrual bleeding. No backup method needed • Can also start immediately or at any other time if it is reasonably certain that she is not pregnant. Use backup method for the next 7 days
Switching from an IUD (including hormonal)	• Start pills within 5 days of start of menrtual bleeding, no additional contraceptive needed & IUD can be removed at that time • Start pills at any other time if it is reasonably certain she is not pregnant. If sexually active in this menstrual cycle and more than 5 days since menstrual bleeding started, remove IUD at time of next menstrual period
After taking ECPs	• Day after ECP** • First day of next menses } if using other interim • Sunday of next menses** } method until menses

* World Health Organization. Selected Practice Recommendations for Contraceptive Use. 2002 ◄
** Back-up method needed until 7 days after starting COCs if it has been more than 5 days since menstrual bleeding started

Figure 26.2

CHOOSING A PILL

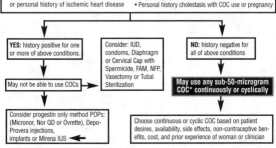

Woman wants to use "the Pill"
Does she have problem of:
- Smoking & age 35 or older
- Moderate or severe hypertension (more than 160/100) (See appendix, A-3)
- Undiagnosed abnormal vaginal bleeding
- Diabetes with vascular complications or more than 20 years duration
- DVT or PE (unless anticoagulated) or current or personal history of ischemic heart disease

- Headaches with focal neurological symptoms or personal history of stroke
- Family history of thrombosis (multiple members, multiple episodes of unexplained venous thromboembolism)
- Current or personal history of breast cancer
- Active viral hepatitis or mild or severe cirrhosis
- Breast-feeding exclusively at the present time
- Major surgery with immobilization within 1 month
- Personal history cholestasis with COC use or pregnancy

YES: history positive for one or more of above conditions.

Consider: IUD, condoms, Diaphragm or Cervical Cap with Spermicide, FAM, NFP, Vasectomy or Tubal Sterilization

NO: history negative for all of above conditions

May not be able to use COCs

May use any sub-50-microgram COC* continuously or cyclically

Consider progestin only method POPs: (Micronor, Nor QD or Ovrette), Depo-Provera injections, implants or Mirena IUS

Choose continuous or cyclic COC based on patient desires, availability, side effects, non-contraceptive benefits, cost, and prior experience of woman or clinician

- The World Health Organization and the Food and Drug Administration both recommend using the **lowest dose pill** that is effective. All combined pills with less than 50 µg of estrogen are effective and safe
- There are no studies demonstrating a decreased risk for deep vein thrombosis (DVT) in women on 20-µg pills. Data on higher dose pills have demonstrated that the less the estrogen dose, the lower the risk for DVT
- All COCs lower free testosterone. In the US, only Ortho Tri-Cyclen and Estrostep have FDA labeling indicating it as a treatment of moderate acne vulgaris, based on results of randomized, placebo controlled trials. Other formulations are under study. Class labeling in Canada for all combined pills states that use of pills may improve acne. In Canada only, Ortho Tri-Cyclen has "treatment of moderate acne vulgaris" as an indication for use
- To minimize discontinuation due to spotting and breakthrough bleeding, warn women in advance, reassure that spotting and breakthrough bleeding become better over time. (See Figure 26.3, p. 107)
- To attain the most favorable lipid profile, consider norgestimate, desogestrel pill or low dose norethindrone acetate, or lowest dose norethindrone (Ovcon-35, Brevicon, Modicon) or ethindiol diacetate (Demulen 1/35 or Zovia 35). No clinical benefits have been demonstrated to be attributable to differences in lipids caused by these pills. Estrogen has a beneficial effect on the walls of blood vessels. All currently available COCs raise triglycerides.

*The package insert for women on Yasmin states *[Berlex-2001]*: "Yasmin is different from other birth control pills because it contains the progestin drospirenone. Drospirenone may increase potassium. Therefore, you should not take Yasmin if you have kidney, liver or adrenal disease, because this could cause serious heart and health problems. Other drugs may also increase potassium. If you are currently on daily, long-term treatment for a chronic condition with any of the medications below, you should consult your healthcare provider about whether Yasmin is right for you, and during the first month that you take Yasmin, you should have a blood test to check your potassium level: NSAIDs (ibuprofen [Motrin®, Advil®], naproxen [Naprosyn®, Aleve®, and others] when taken long-term and daily for treatment of arthritis or other problems]; potassium-sparing diuretics (sprironolactone and others); potassium supplementation; ACE inhibitors (Capoten®, Vasotec®, Zestril® and others); Angiotensin-II receptor antagonists (Cozaar®, Diovan®, Avapro® and others); heparin"

Figure 26.3

SPOTTING/BREAKTHROUGH BLEEDING ON COCs

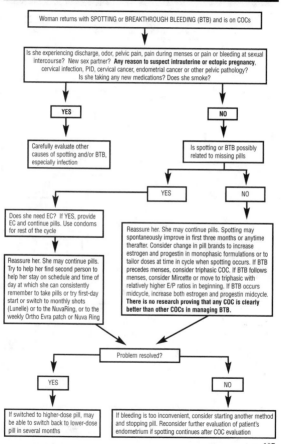

Woman returns with SPOTTING or BREAKTHROUGH BLEEDING (BTB) and is on COCs

↓

Is she experiencing discharge, odor, pelvic pain, pain during menses or pain or bleeding at sexual intercourse? New sex partner? **Any reason to suspect intrauterine or ectopic pregnancy,** cervical infection, PID, cervical cancer, endometrial cancer or other pelvic pathology? Is she taking any new medications? Does she smoke?

YES → Carefully evaluate other causes of spotting and/or BTB, especially infection

NO → Is spotting or BTB possibly related to missing pills

YES →

Does she need EC? If YES, provide EC and continue pills. Use condoms for rest of the cycle

Reassure her. She may continue pills. Try to help her find second person to help her stay on schedule and time of day at which she can consistently remember to take pills or try first-day start or switch to monthly shots (Lunelle) or to the NuvaRing, or to the weekly Ortho Evra patch or Nuva Ring

NO →

Reassure her. She may continue pills. Spotting may spontaneously improve in first three months or anytime thereafter. Consider change in pill brands to increase estrogen and progestin in monophasic formulations or to tailor doses at time in cycle when spotting occurs. If BTB precedes menses, consider triphasic COC. If BTB follows menses, consider Mircette or move to triphasic with relatively higher E/P ratios in beginning. If BTB occurs midcycle, increase both estrogen and progestin midcycle. **There is no research proving that any COC is clearly better than other COCs in managing BTB.**

↓

Problem resolved?

YES → If switched to higher-dose pill, may be able to switch back to lower-dose pill in several months

NO → If bleeding is too inconvenient, consider starting another method and stopping pill. Reconsider further evaluation of patient's endometrium if spotting continues after COC evaluation

Figure 26.4

NEW ONSET OR WORSENING HEADACHES IN COC USERS

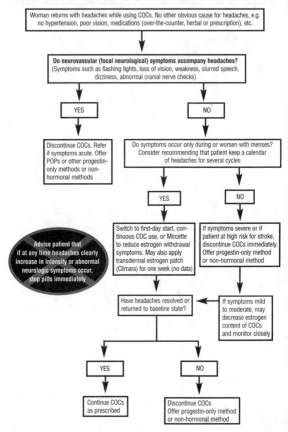

Woman returns with headaches while using COCs. No other obvious cause for headaches, e.g. no hypertension, poor vision, medications (over-the-counter, herbal or prescription), etc.

Do neurovascular (focal neurological) symptoms accompany headaches?
(Symptoms such as flashing lights, loss of vision, weakness, slurred speech, dizziness, abnormal cranial nerve checks)

YES

NO

Discontinue COCs. Refer if symptoms acute. Offer POPs or other progestin-only methods or non-hormonal methods

Do symptoms occur only during or worsen with menses? Consider recommending that patient keep a calendar of headaches for several cycles

YES

NO

Switch to first-day start, continuous COC use, or Mircette to reduce estrogen withdrawal symptoms. May also apply transdermal estrogen patch (Climara) for one week (no data)

If symptoms severe or if patient at high risk for stroke, discontinue COCs immediately. Offer progestin-only method or non-hormonal method

Advise patient that if at any time headaches clearly increase in intensity or abnormal neurologic symptoms occur, stop pills immediately

Have headaches resolved or returned to baseline state?

If symptoms mild to moderate, may decrease estrogen content of COCs and monitor closely

YES

NO

Continue COCs as prescribed

Discontinue COCs. Offer progestin-only method or non-hormonal method

Figure 26.5

MAKING THE TRANSITION FROM COCs TO MENOPAUSE, WITH OR WITHOUT HORMONE THERAPY (HT)

The transition from COCs to menopause, with or without HT may be accomplished in a number of ways. Some reviewers of this algorithm switch to a 20 or 25-mcg pill if the patient is going to use COCs into the early 50s. Certainly a major concern must be unintended pregnancy. Work together to determine a method for pregnancy prevention that is acceptable and effective

This algorithm does NOT include testing for a woman's menopausal status using FSH or LH tests*

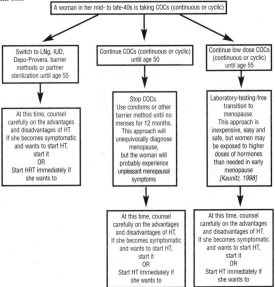

*FSH and LH testing are problematic because they show current status only. A perimenopausal woman can seem to be menopausal according to lab tests but ovulate unpredictably after that.

DESCRIPTION: One Ortho Evra patch is worn for one week for each of 3 consecutive weeks, usually on the lower abdomen or buttocks. It can also be applied to the upper outer arm or to the upper torso (except for the breasts). The fourth week is patch-free to permit withdrawal bleeding this week the woman has her period. This 4.5 cm square patch delivers 20 micrograms of ethinyl estradiol and 150 mcg of the progestin, norelgestromin (the active metabolite of norgestimate) daily. *[Grimes-2001]* It takes 2 days to achieve steady states or plateau levels of hormones after application of the patch

MECHANISM: The patch prevents pregnancy in the same ways that combined pills do

COST: The patch costs approximately the same as one cycle of pills

EFFECTIVENESS

Among *perfect* users (users who apply transdermal contraceptive patches on schedule and each patch remains in place for the full week), only 3-6 in 1,000 women (0.3-0.6%) are expected to become pregnant during the first year (Table 13.2 on p. 38). Pooled data from three contraceptive efficacy studies (22,155 treatment cycles) using life table analysis found an overall failure rate of about 1% (0.8% or 8 pregnancies per 1000 women through 13 cycles). *[Zieman-2001]*

In a multicenter trial of 1417 women randomized to use the patch (n=812) or the oral contraceptive, Triphasil (n=605), the pregnancy rate was lower (but not significantly lower) with the patch than with the pills. There were 5 pregnancies among women using the patch (1 user failure and 4 method failures). *[Audet-2001]* Of 15 pregnancies in the 3 clinical trials of the Ortho Evra Patch, 5 were in women who were markedly overweight (women more than 90 kilograms or 198 pounds). *[Zieman-2001]* In an open-label study of 1,672 women receiving the Ortho Evra patch for 6 or 13 cycles, 6 pregnancies occurred, and 4 of them were in women weighing 90 kg or more *[Smallwood-2001]*. There are no data available about typical failure rates. Correct and consistent use was significantly better among patch users compared to pill users

ADVANTAGES

Menstrual: Like combined pills

Sexual/Psychological:
- May enhance sexual enjoyment due to diminished fear of pregnancy
- Nothing to do on a daily basis (ideal for women who forget to take pills) ◄—
- Does not interrupt intercourse

Cancers/tumors and masses: No data yet; benefits probably quite comparable to combined pills

Other:
- Option throughout the reproductive years: Age is not a reason to avoid the Patch. For some women compliance may be easier than taking a pill every day *[Audet-2001]*. Each patch ◄— contains enough hormone to suppress ovulation for up to 9 days. In randomized trials compliance was perfect in 88.2% of participants' cycles, significantly better than in women taking pills (in 77.7% of women's cycles on pills compliance was perfect). *[Audet 2001]*
- Although there are no data yet, Ortho Evra may be used as are continuous OCPs - e.g. for 9 weeks in a row then a 7 day patch-free interval *[Guillebaud-Personal communication 10/14/01]*

DISADVANTAGES

Menstrual: In the first cycle about one-fifth of patch users experienced breakthrough bleeding or spotting. There were no statistically significant differences between the patch and COCs with regard to breakthrough bleeding in any cycle in the randomized trial of the patch vs Triphasil. *[Audet 2001]*

Sexual/Psychological: See page 95

Cancers/tumors and masses: None

Other:
- Lack of protection against sexually transmitted infections (STIs)
- Among 812 women on the patch, 3 serious adverse events were considered possible or likely related to use of the patch, including 1 case of pain and paraesthesia in the left arm, 1 case of migraine and 1 case of cholecystitis *[Audet-2001]*
- Must remove and replace patch weekly. Application site problems include partial detachment (2.8%) or complete detachment (1.8%) and skin irritation (1.1%) *[Audet-2001]*. Hyperpigmentation has been noted under the site of patch application. In a study of patch wear under conditions of physical exertion and variable temperatures and humidity, less than 2% of patches were replaced for complete or partial detachment. 2.6% of women discontinued using the patch because of application site reactions. Problems did not increase over time *[Audet-2001]*. Border of patch may become dirty, picking up lint, hairs or fabric

COMPLICATIONS
- Nausea occurred in 20.4% of women on patch vs 18.3% of women using oral contraceptives; patch was discontinued by 1.8% of women because of nausea. *[Audet-2001]*
- Breast discomfort was greater in women using the patch than in women on the pill. The difference was significant only in cycles 1 and 2 (15.4% vs 3.5% in cycle 1 and 6.6% vs. 1.5% in cycle 2). For cycles 3-13, breast discomfort occurred in 0 to 3.2% of women using the patch and in 0 to 1.7% of women on pills (not statistically significant). *[Audet-2001]*
- Headaches were as likely in women on patch (21.9%) as in women on pills (22.1%)

PRESCRIBING PRECAUTIONS
- Precautions for the patch are the same as those for combined pills (see page 98)
- **Women weighing more than 90 kg (198 lbs)** should be told that the patch may be slightly less effective and that they should consider using a backup

CANDIDATES FOR USE
- Women wanting to avoid having something to do every day, or at the time of intercourse
- Women wanting regular menstrual periods. May be used by individuals allergic to latex
- **Adolescents:** **Excellent option, particularly for teenage women unable to remember to take pills daily** *[Archer-2002]*

INITIATING METHOD:
- With the 1st pack of patches, the patient is eligible for up to three free replacement patches. Write prescription for "replacement patch" with the first box of patches
- **A pelvic examination is not necessary prior to starting this method** *[Stewart-2001]*
- Ask patient, "What day of the week is the easiest for you to remember?" and start then
- It is usually recommended that the first patch be placed on the first day of the next menstrual period. If started any other day use a backup contraceptive for 7 days
- Women switching from pills should start on first day of menses. Do not wait to complete pack of pills
- Women switching from DMPA should start about 2 days before next injection is due
- But as with pills, the patch can be started anytime with backup for 7 days, if you are reasonably sure the woman is not pregnant

INSTRUCTIONS FOR PATIENT
- If the PATCH-FREE interval is more than 9 days (late restart), apply a new patch and use backup contraception for 7 days
- No band-aids, tatoos, or decals on top of patch as this might alter absorption of hormones
- Smooth the edges down when you first put it on
- Avoid placing patch on exactly the same site 2 consecutive weeks
- Location of patch should not be altered in mid-week
- Women should check the patch daily to make sure all edges remain closely adherent to skin
- Single replacement patches are available through pharmacists. The manufacturer will reimburse a woman for up to $12 for the replacement patch

FOLLOW UP

- What is happening to your menstrual periods?
- Have you experienced skin irritation?
- Has your patch ever come off partially or completely?
- Have you had problems remembering to replace your patch each week for 3 weeks followed by a week of no patch?
- Do you plan to have children? OR Do you plan to have more children?

FERTILITY AFTER USE: Likely the same excellent return of fertility as COCs

INJECTIONS – MONTHLY – LUNELLE

DESCRIPTION: Lunelle is a 0.5 cc suspension containing 25 mg medroxyprogesterone acetate and 5 mg estradiol cypionate injected intramuscularly into the deltoid or gluteus maximus muscle every 28 ± 5 days (ideally every 28-30 days). Estradiol cypionate is metabolized to estradiol in the bloodstream. Brand names: Lunelle, Lunella, Cylco-Provera, Cyclofem, Ciclofemina, Feminena and HRP 112. More information is available to clinicians from Pharmacia by calling 1-800-253-8600 ext. 38244. It is possible that Lunelle will ◄ never return as an option

MECHANISM: Same as COCs; primary mechanism is suppression of ovulation

EFFECTIVENESS
Perfect use failure rate in first year: 0.05%
Typical use failure rate in first year: 3% *[Trussel J IN Contraceptive Technology-2003]*

COST: Price of drug is similar to brand-name COCs. Price of administration of drug may vary. Health departments in the State of Washington pay 11 times more for an injection of Lunelle, $16.66, as they pay for the average cycle of pills, $1.35 *[Margulies-2001]*

ADVANTAGES
Menstrual:
- Excellent cycle control after first few cycles
- Decreases ovulatory pain (Mittelschmerz) and dysmenorrhea
- Prevents internal hemorrhage from ovulation in women with coagulation defects
- Prevents hemorrhagic corpus luteum cysts
- Combined injectable users are less likely to experience bleeding pattern changes than users of progestin-only injectables *[Hall-1998]*

Sexual/psychological:
- May enhance sexual enjoyment due to diminished fear of pregnancy
- Convenient: one injection provides up to 33 days protection. No disruption at time of intercourse; facilitates spontaneity

Cancers/tumors & masses: No documented effects, but probably similar to protective effects of COCs

Other:
- 10 day window of time 28 ± 5 days (ideally every 28-30 days) over which injections may be given (flexibility!) In average woman, ovulation on Lunelle actually is suppressed for about 40 days which is more than 28 + 5 days
- Effective, convenient, rapidly reversible, & private *[Hall-1998][Kaunitz-1999][Shulman-1999]*
- May diminish adverse effects on triglycerides seen with COCs (no clinically demonstrated benefits as of the present time)
- Less effect on clotting factors than COCs; No clotting or cardiovascular complications in WHO studies
- Self-injection is a possibility and pharmacists will give Lunelle injecitons in some states ◄

DISADVANTAGES

Menstrual: First period usually comes 2-3 weeks after first injection of Lunelle
- Increased number of days of spotting/bleeding in first month of use. Excessive bleeding in some women. Then predictable pattern established with bleeding every month, 2-3 weeks after injection
- Amenorrhea in 1% (first cycle) to 4% (60th week) of cycles. In cycles 2-12, 15% of Lunelle users experienced a missed period *[Kaunitz-1999]*

Sexual/psychological:
- Depression, anxiety, irritability, fatigue, other mood changes or decreased interest in sexual intercourse may develop (same as COCs)
- Fear of needles may preclude use of this method

Cancers/ tumors and masses: No documented impact

Other:
- Must return each month for reinjection (every 28 ± 5 days); Doesn't have to return if she has a friend or school nurse to administer shots. May be confused with the 13-week/3 month regimen called Depo-Provera. The manufacturer, Pharmacia, is developing a system to remind Lunelle users each month that their Lunelle injections are due
- The annual cost of the medication and injection may exceed the cost of other reversible contraceptives
- Weight gain in one year (median values: 2-4 lbs. in women ≤ 150 lbs.; 2-6 lbs. in women > 150 lbs.) *[Kaunitz-1999]* Weight gain was the leading cause of method-related discontinuation in U.S. trials
- If side effects develop, a woman must wait 4-6 weeks for symptoms to subside
- No protection against STIs; must use condoms if at risk
- Mastalgia reported and other hormonal side effects

COMPLICATIONS: Inflammation of the injection site may occur

PRESCRIBING PRECAUTIONS: *Same as COCs; Package labeling same as COCs*
(see WHO Criteria, pages A-1 – A-8)
- Known or suspected pregnancy
- Less than three weeks postpartum because of increased DVT risk (WHO: 3)
- Breastfeeding and less than six weeks postpartum (WHO: 4)
- Thrombophlebitis or thromboembolic disorder; history of DVT or VTE disorders
- Hypertension or with vascular disease ⟶ 140-159 = 3 (WHO) ≥160 = 4 (WHO)
                                                      90-99 ≥100
- Cerebral vascular or coronary artery disease
- Diabetes with vascular involvement or > 20 years duration ⟵
- Undiagnosed abnormal vaginal bleeding (WHO: 2)
- Liver dysfunction or disease such as hepatic adenoma or carcinoma; history of cholestatic jaundice of pregnancy or jaundice with prior hormonal contraceptive use
- Valvular heart disease with complications or ischemic heart disease ⟵
- Estrogen dependent neoplasm including breast cancer
- Headaches with focal neurologic symptoms
- Known hypersensitivity to ingredients
- Smoking over age 35

CANDIDATES FOR USE
- Women who are candidates for estrogen/progestin combined hormonal medication and who:
  1. Do not want to have to remember to take a pill daily and desire greater efficacy than pills
  2. Appreciate convenience of injections and desire more regular menses than with DMPA

3. Have had bleeding irregularities or weight gain on DMPA or Norplant
4. Want private method

DRUG INTERACTIONS: Unknown, but may be similar to COCs
• Aminoglutethimide may decrease serum medroxyprogesterone acetate

INITIATING METHOD
• **A pelvic examination is not necessary to initiate this method** *[Stewart-2001]*
• First injection is to be given in first 5 days after onset of menses, within 10 days of an abortion or 4 weeks postpartum (unless breastfeeding)
• Could also be given at other time in cycle if reasonably certain patient is not pregnant
  If given at other times, recommend backup for 7 days
• If switching from DMPA give when next injection is due (no backup) ◄—

INSTRUCTIONS FOR PATIENT
• No backup method needed if started within 5 days of menses
• Expect first menses early (approximately 2 weeks after injection)
• At each visit, provide oral and written date of next injection based on 28 ± 5 days (eg ◄— come back July 20 ± 5 days). Give appointment
• Each subsequent menses depends on timing of previous injection

FOLLOW-UP
• What is happening to your menstrual periods?
• Have you had pain at the injection site?
• Have you gained 5 lbs. or more? (see WEIGHT GAIN, A TEACHABLE MOMENT p. 125)
• Have you had the feeling that you might be pregnant?
• Are you having problems returning on time for injections?
• Do you plan to have children? OR Do you plan to have more children?

PROBLEM MANAGEMENT
• Similar to COCs
• If a woman has heavy or prolonged menses, injection of Lunelle after just 21-23 days may decrease bleeding
• If there is pain or infection at injection site see p. 126

FERTILITY AFTER USE
• Excellent return to baseline fertility: 2 month delay from last injection
• Fertility returns considerably faster than with Depo-Provera; five months after the last Lunelle injection, nearly twice as many users are able to conceive compared to women using Depo-Provera *[Kaunitz -1999]*

VAGINAL CONTRACEPTIVE RING – MONTHLY – NuvaRing

DESCRIPTION: (also see www.nuvaring.com) The NuvaRing is a combined hormonal contraceptive consisting of a 5.4 cm (2 inches) diameter flexible ring, 4 mm (1/8 inch) in thickness. The ring is made of ethylene vinylacetate polymer. It is left in place in the vagina for 3 weeks and then removed for a week to allow withdrawal bleeding. **It is not necessary that the ring be removed for intercourse; it is generally recommended that it not be removed for intercourse.** Douching is discouraged but topical therapies are allowed. NuvaRing releases low doses of ethinyl estradiol (15 micrograms daily) and etonogestrel, the active form of desogestrel (120 micrograms daily). With oral hormones there is a daily spike in hormone levels after the woman swallows each dose, followed by a gradual drop throughout the rest of the day. A single vaginal ring maintains a steady, low release rate while in place

MECHANISM

- This method suppresses ovulation *[Mulders-2001]*. In one study, ovulation is suppressed ◀ for 39 days
- Other contraceptive effects similar to combined pills

COST: Each ring will cost approximately the same as one cycle of pills

EFFECTIVENESS

- Overall pregnancy rate of 0.3 *[Trussell-2004]* to 0.65 *[Roumen-2001]* per 100 woman-years ◀ (all first-year users)

ADVANTAGES

Menstrual:
- Withdrawal bleeding occurs in 98% of cycles, and bleeding at other times in only 6.4% of cycles *[Roumen-2001]*; better withdrawal/spotting pattern than COCs probably due to ◀ NOT forgetting pills and the steady even blood levels that are achieved
- Irregular bleeding is low in the first cycle of use (less than 5%) and continues to be low throughout subsequent cycles *[Roumen-2001]*

Sexual/Psychological: Decreased fear of pregnancy may increase pleasure from intercourse
Cancers/tumors and masses: No published data; probably similar to COCs
Other: There are only 2 tasks for ring users to remember: insertion and removal once a month
- 95% of women say they cannot feel it
- 70% of partners say they cannot feel it
- The lowest dose combined estrogen and progestin method ◀
- Privacy - no visible patch or pill packages ◀

DISADVANTAGES

Menstrual
- Withdrawal bleeding continued beyond the ring-free interval in about one quarter of cycles (20% to 27%) *[Roumen-2001]*. However, most of the time it is just spotting

Sexual/Psychological: Some women dislike placing/removing objects into/out of vagina ◀
Cancers/tumors and masses: None
Other: **Table 26.3 Adverse Events Reported by Vaginal Contraceptive Ring Users**

Adverse event *	Related** (%)	Total (%)
Headache	6.6	11.8
Nausea	2.8	4.5
Weight increase	2.2	3.0
Breast pain	1.9	2.8
Dysmenorrhea	1.8	2.6
Depression	1.7	2.4
Leukorrhea	5.3	5.9 ◀
Vaginitis	5.0	13.7 ◀
Device related events***	3.8	4.1 ◀
Vaginal discomfort	2.2	2.4 ◀

* Adverse events occurring in 1% or more of the 1,145 treated subjects
** Possibly, probably or definitely treatment-related as judged by investigator
***Foreign body sensation, coital problems, device expulsion

Source: Adapted from Table IV Incidence of adverse events. Roumen FJME, Apter D, Mulders TMT, et al. Efficacy, tolerability and acceptability of a novel contraceptive vaginal ring releasing etonogestrel and ethinyl oestradiol. Human Reproduction 2001; 16:469-475.

COMPLICATIONS: See Table 26.2, page 113

PRESCRIBING PRECAUTIONS
• The WHO Medical Eligibility Criteria for the NuvaRing are the same as for combined pills
• Women who are hesitant about touching their genitalia or who have difficulty inserting ◀
  or removing ring

CANDIDATES FOR USE
• Women wanting to avoid having something to remember to do every day, or at the time of
  intercourse
• Women wanting regular menstrual periods
Adolescents: Excellent option; requires less discipline than taking pills daily

INITIATING METHOD
• A new ring is inserted any time during the first 5 days of a normal menstrual cycle
• New ring can be inserted at any time in cycle if reasonably certain woman is not ◀
  pregnant; use backup x 7 days

INSTRUCTIONS FOR PATIENT
• The package insert states that backup must be used during the first 7 days that the ◀
  first ring is in place
• The NuvaRing is removed at the end of 3 weeks of wear; then, after one ring-free week, the
  woman inserts a new ring
• The woman's menstrual period occurs during the ring-free week
• Ring removal during intercourse is **not** recommended; however, women who want to
  remove it during intercourse may do so without having to use a backup method as long as
  it is not removed for longer than 3 hours
• No special accuracy is required for ring placement; absorption is fine anywhere in the vagina
• Because the ring is small and flexible, most women do not notice any pressure or discomfort,
  and it is not likely to be uncomfortable for their partners during intercourse
• Always have 2 rings on hand in case one is lost
• If the ring is left in place longer than three weeks, the user is probably still protected from
  pregnancy for more than 30 days by the same ring. The NuvaRing remains effective for
  beyond 21 days, allowing clinicians flexibility in how often they tell women the ring must
  be replaced. For example, the ring could be reinserted on the first of the month each ◀
  month with no hormone-free interval (similar to taking combined pills with no hormone-
  free days). (Obviously off-label)

FOLLOW UP: Similar to women on pills; ask about difficulty during removal or insertion.
Women may need closer follow-up if they have:
• genital prolapse
• severe constipation
• frequent vaginal infection (i.e. recurrent yeast infection)

FERTILITY AFTER USE: Presumably excellent but no data yet

PILLS - DAILY - often called MINI-PILLS

DESCRIPTION

Progestin-only pills (POPs) are also known as mini-pills. POPs contain only a progestin and are taken daily with no hormone-free days. POPs have lower progestin doses than combined pills. Each tablet of Micronor and Nor-QD contains 0.35 mg norethindrone. Each tablet of Ovrette has 0.075 mg of norgestrel.

EFFECTIVENESS [Trussell J IN Contraceptive Technology 2004]
Perfect use failure rate in first year: 0.3% (See Table 13.2, p. 38) ◄
(if 200 women take POPs for 1 year, only 1 will become pregnant in the first year of perfect use)
Typical use failure rate in first year: 8.0% ◄

MECHANISM

Thickens cervical mucus to prevent sperm entry into upper reproductive tract (major mechanism). Effect short lived - requires punctual dosing. Other mechanisms include ovulation suppression (in about 50% of cycles), thin, atrophic endometrium which inhibits implantation; and slowed tubal mobility

COST [Trussell, 1995; Smith, 1993]
• POPs cost more than combined pills both in pharmacies and in sales to public programs

ADVANTAGES
Menstrual:
• Decreased menstrual blood loss, cramps and pain, amenorrhea (10% of women). Amenorrhea is more likely with punctual dosing ◄
• Decrease in ovulatory pain (Mittelschmerz) in cycles when ovulation suppressed
Sexual/physiological:
• May enhance sexual enjoyment due to diminished fear of pregnancy
• No disruption at time of intercourse; facilitates spontaneity
Cancers, tumors and masses:
• Possible protection against endometrial cancer
Other:
• Rapid return to baseline fertility
• Possible reduction in PID risk due to cervical mucus thickening
• Good option for women who cannot use estrogen but want to take pills
• May be used by smokers over age 35. **Discourage smoking, of course!** ◄
• May be used by breastfeeding women. Discontinue if production of milk decreases ◄

DISADVANTAGES
Menstrual:
• Irregular menses ranging from amenorrhea to increased days of spotting and bleeding but with reduced blood loss overall

Sexual/psychological:
- Spotting and bleeding may interfere with sexual activity
- Intermittent amenorrhea may raise concerns about pregnancy
- Possible increase in depression, anxiety, irritability, fatigue or other mood changes, but often POPs reduce risk of these disorders

Cancers, tumors and masses:
- May be associated with slightly higher risk of persistent ovarian follicles

Other:
- Must take pill at same time each day (more than 3-hour delay considered by some clinicians to be equivalent to a "missed pill")
- Effect on cervical mucus decreases after 22 hours and is gone after 27 hours
- No protection against STIs

COMPLICATIONS
- Allergy to progestin pill is rare
- Amenorrheic, Latina, breast-feeding women who had gestational diabetes may be at higher risk of developing overt diabetes in first year postpartum *[Kjos, 1998]*

CANDIDATES FOR USE (see Year 2000 WHO Medical Eligibility Criteria, A-1 - A-8)
- Virtually every woman who can take pills on a daily basis can be a candidate for POPs,
- POPs are particularly good for women with contraindications to or side effects from estrogen or higher-dose progestins:
  - Women with personal history of thrombosis or strong family history of VTE
  - Recently postpartum women
  - Women who are exclusively breast-feeding
  - Smokers over age 35
  - Women who had or fear chloasma, worsening migraine headaches, hypertriglyceridemia or other estrogen-related side effects
  - Women with hypertension, coronary artery disease or cerebrovascular disease (see WHO Precautions in Appendix)

PRESCRIBING PRECAUTIONS
Progestin-only pills can be used by all women willing and able to take daily pills except:
- Suspected or demonstrated pregnancy (although there are no proven harmful effects for the fetus)
- Current breast cancer or less than 5 years ago (WHO:3) ←
- Hepatic failure, jaundice
- Inability to absorb sex steroids from gastrointestinal tract (active colitis, etc.)
- Taking medications that increase hepatic clearance (rifampin, certain anticonvulsants, St. Johns Wort or griseofulvin). Efficacy in combination with Orlistat and other fat-binding agents is not well studied
- Conditions contributing to noncompliance

MEDICAL ELIGIBILITY CHECKLIST: Ask the client the questions below. If she answers NO to ALL of the questions, then she CAN use POPs if she wants. If she answers YES to a question below, follow the instructions; in some cases she can still use POPs

1. Do you think you are pregnant?

☐ No ☐ Yes Assess if pregnant. If she might be pregnant, give her condoms or spermicide to use until reasonably sure that she is not pregnant. Then she can start POPs

2. Do you have or have you ever had breast cancer? (See page A4)

☐ No ☐ Yes Do not provide POPs. Help her choose a method without hormones

3. Do you have jaundice, severe cirrhosis of the liver, acute liver infection or tumor? (Are her eyes or skin unusually yellow?) (See page A5)

☐ No ☐ Yes Perform physical exam and arrange lab tests or refer. If she has serious active liver disease (jaundice, painful or enlarged liver, viral hepatitis, liver tumor), do not provide POPs. Refer for care. Help her choose a method without hormones

4. Do you have vaginal bleeding that is unusual for you? (See page A3)

☐ No ☐ Yes If she is not pregnant but has unexplained vaginal bleeding that suggests an underlying medical condition, can provide POPs since neither the underlying condition nor its assessment will be affected. Assess and treat any underlying condition as appropriate, or refer. Reassess POP use based on findings

5. Are you taking medicine for seizures? Taking rifampin (rifampicin), griseofulvin or aminoglutethimide? St. Johns Wort?

☐ No ☐ Yes If she is taking phenytoin, carbamazepine, barbiturate, or primidone for seizures or rifampin, griseofulvin, aminoglutethamide or St. John's Wort, provide condoms or spermicide or help her choose another method that is more effective, such as DMPA. Use of valproic acid does NOT lower the effectiveness of POPs. Discuss ECPs

6. Do you have problems with severe diarrhea from Crohn's disease or other bowel disorders? Or are you using medications that block fat absorption?

☐ No ☐ Yes Help her choose a non-oral method of birth control

7. If patient < 1 year since delivering and had gestational diabetes, ask if she is breast-feeding?

☐ No ☐ Yes Counsel that she may be at higher risk for developing glucose ◄— intolerance if she remains amenorrheic. Consider IUD or COCs, if feasible

SPECIAL SITUATIONS

History of pregnancy while using POPs correctly:
- Consider DMPA or switch to estrogen containing methods or IUDs
- Continue POPs but add condoms or other backup with every act of coitus

Use with a broad-spectrum antibiotic such as tetracycline or erythromycin:
- Few studies support antibiotic's role in contraceptive failure. Some clinicians encourage backup for first 1-2 weeks, others for full duration of antibiotic use. Explain conflicting advice now being given; let patient decide whether to use backup method.
  Go to: www.managingcontraception.com/questions_new/oral/g-a_or_06-12.html

INITIATING METHOD

• **A pelvic examination is not necessary prior to initiation of this method**
• *New starts:* Offer condoms either for back-up for 7 days or for use should patient stop
  POPs. Also offer advance prescription of PLAN B or give her a package of PLAN B
• *Post-partum:* May initiate immediately regardless of breast-feeding status (PPFA, UCSF,
  Grady Memorial Hospital)
  Note: WHO and IPPF are concerned about hypothetical impact of POPs on breast milk
  production and recommend waiting until at least 6 weeks to initiate use of DMPA and POPs ◄
• *After miscarriage or abortion:* Start immediately
• *Menstruating women:* Start on menses if possible. May initiate anytime in cycle if woman
  is not pregnant, but recommend at least 1-week back-up barrier method
• *Switching from IUD, COCs, DMPA, to POPs:* start immediately. Need for back-up depends
  on previous method used: **IUD:** start immediately, backup for 7 days; Some clinicians say
  48 hours minimum; others say no backup. **COCs:** start immediately if cycle of hormonally
  active pills completed; backup not necessary if no pill-free interval. **DMPA:** start
  immediately if switching at or before next DMPA injection due (no backup necessary)

INSTRUCTIONS FOR PATIENT

• Take one pill daily at *same* time each day until end of pack. Start next pack the next day
• If at risk for infection, use condoms with every act of intercourse
• If you miss a pill by more than 3 hours from regular time, take the missed pill(s) and use
  backup for 48 hours. Consider using emergency contraception if sex in past 3-5 days

FOLLOW-UP

• How many pills do you typically miss or are late taking per week? Per pack?
• Have you missed any pills in last 3 days? (candidate for EC)
• Have you missed any periods or experienced any symptoms of pregnancy?
• What has your menstrual bleeding been like?
• Have you had any increase in headaches, depression or change in vision?
• Do you plan to have children? OR Do you plan to have more children?
• What are you doing to protect yourself from STIs? ◄

PROBLEM MANAGEMENT

• *Amenorrhea:* Rule out pregnancy with first episode or whenever symptoms of pregnancy
  noted. Otherwise, amenorrhea is not harmful when women take progestin-only pills
• *Irregular bleeding:* After finding out if missing pills, rule out STIs, pregnancy, cancer. If
  not at risk and no evidence of underlying pathology, reassure patient; 3-day course of high
  dose NSAIDS may help
• *Heavy bleeding:* Rule out STIs, pregnancy, cancer. If no evidence of underlying pathology,
  rule out clinically significant anemia. Trial of 3 days high dose NSAIDS. If fails, may need
  estrogen-containing contraceptives (addition of physiologic doses ERT only may
  compromise cervical mucus barrier) or other non-hormonal methods of contraception
• *Abdominal pain:* Consider pelvic pathology (ectopic pregnancy, torsion, PID) and refer
  for treatment. If ovarian cyst is cause, it may be managed conservatively. Progestin slows
  follicular atresia. Recheck in 6 weeks and anytime her symptoms worsen
• *Severe headaches:* If new onset or worsening of headaches, blurred vision with flashing
  lights, loss of vision, trouble moving or speaking - stop POPs and seek immediate help.
  Offer nonhormonal contraceptive

FERTILITY AFTER USE: Fertility returns to its baseline levels promptly

DMPA INJECTIONS (DEPO-PROVERA)

DESCRIPTION: 1 cc of a crystalline suspension of 150 mg depot medroxyprogesterone acetate injected intramuscularly into the deltoid or gluteus maximus muscle every 11-13 weeks For more information, call 1-800-253-8600 ext. 38244

EFFECTIVENESS *[Trussell J IN Contraceptive Technology - 2004]*
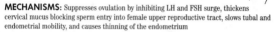
• Approved labeling indicates each injection effective for up to 13 weeks
Perfect use failure rate in first year: 0.3% (See Table 13.2, p. 38) ◄
Typical use failure rate in first year: 3% ◄
Continuation at 1 year: 42% *[Polaneczky-1996]* - 56% *[Trussell-2004]* ◄

MECHANISMS: Suppresses ovulation by inhibiting LH and FSH surge, thickens cervical mucus blocking sperm entry into female upper reproductive tract, slows tubal and endometrial mobility, and causes thinning of the endometrium

COST: In Washington State, health departments pay $4.75 for 28 days of contraception for a woman receiving Depo-Provera each 3 months. This is 4 times greater than the cost of pills for the same clinics, $1.35 per cycle. *[Margulies - 2001]* In 2001, the price at these same clinics for the new one-month injectable, Lunelle, was $16.66 per monthly cycle

ADVANTAGES
Menstrual:

• Less menstrual blood loss, anemia, or hemorrhagic corpus luteum cysts
• After 1 year of use, 50% of women develop amenorrhea; 80% develop amenorrhea in 5 years. For this to be an advantage, it must be explained well at first and subsequent visits. See discussion of structured counseling on page 14 ◄
• Decreased menstrual cramps, pain and ovulation pain
• Possible improvement in endometriosis

Sexual/psychological:

• Intercourse may be more pleasurable without worry of pregnancy
• Convenient: permits spontaneous sexual activity; requires no action at time of intercourse

Cancers, tumors, and masses:

• Significant reduction in risk of endometrial cancer
• Possible reduction in risk of ovarian cancer (several studies have failed to show a protective effect)

Benefits for women with medical problems:

• Suppresses ovulation, bleeding and menstrual blood loss in anticoagulated women and women with bleeding diathesis; decreases anemia
• Reduces acute sickle cell crises by 70% *[de Abood-1997]* ◄
• Best method for women on anticonvulsant drugs; may actually decrease seizures and effectiveness not compromised
• Amenorrhea and prolonged effective contraception may be very important for severely developmentally or physically challenged women. One reviewer makes home visits for ◄ some wheelchair bound patients who love Depo-Provera
• Possible improvement of endometriosis

Other:

• The drop in teen pregnancies in 1990s, abortions and births, is attributed to Depo-Provera, Norplant, EC and condoms
• Significantly reduces risk for ectopic pregnancies and may slightly decrease risk of PID
• Convenient: single injection provides at least 13 weeks protection

- Most protocols call for administration anytime between 11 and 13 weeks. However, DMPA is usually forgiving of late injections and is effective in many women for more than 13 weeks (patients should not count on this)
- Less user-dependent than POPs, COCs
- Good option for women who cannot use estrogen (see CANDIDATES FOR USE)
- Private: no visible clue that patient is using; no one else needs to know
- May be used by nursing mothers

DISADVANTAGES

Menstrual:
- Irregular menses during first several months: many women experience unpredictable spotting and bleeding, occasionally blood loss reported to be heavy but unlikely to cause anemia. After 6-12 months, amenorrhea more likely (50% after 1 year)

Sexual/psychological: Also see weight gain, below
- Spotting and bleeding may interfere with sexual activity
- Amenorrhea may raise patient's fears of pregnancy or build-up of menses in uterus if not explained well
- Hypoestrogenism can (infrequently) cause dyspareunia, hot flashes or decreased libido
- Possible increase in depression, anxiety, irritation, PMS, fatigue or other mood changes, but often DMPA reduces risk of these disorders
- Fear of needles may make this an unacceptable choice

Cancers, tumors, and masses: Reduces risk for endometrial hyperplasia and cancer

Other: (See boxed message: Depo Provera & Bones on p. 123)
- No protection against STIs: must use condoms if at risk
- Shedding of HIV may be slightly increased ◄
- Must return every 11-13 weeks for injection
- Long acting: not immediately reversible
- Slow to return to baseline fertility: average 10 months from last injection
- Occasionally, hypoestrogenism ($E_2 < 25$) may develop as a result of FSH suppression. Potential for decreased bone mineral density if used for prolonged period without opportunity for recovery prior to menopause
- Severe headaches may occur
- Acne, hirsutism may develop
- Possible increase in diabetes risk in amenorrheic breastfeeding women with diagnosis of gestational diabetes during first year postpartum [Kjos 1999]
- Metabolic impacts: glucose (slight rise), LDL (slight rise or neutral), HDL (may decrease)
- Other hormone-related Sx: breast tenderness, bloating, hair loss, vasomotor symptoms

COMPLICATIONS

- Progressive significant weight gain. Average of 5.4 lbs in first year and 16.5 lbs after 5 yrs [Schwallie-1973] See boxed message p. 125
- Severe depression (rare) (average MMPI does not change in women on DMPA). Severe crying jags have occurred in women about 1 hour post injection ◄
- Severe allergic reaction, including anaphylaxis (very rare). May consider having women wait in or near office for 20 minutes after injection. (Reviewers disagree about this recommendation, especially for previous DMPA users). Ask patients to report itching ◄ at injection site

CANDIDATES FOR USE (See new (2000) WHO Criteria on pages A-1 through A-8)

- Women who want intermediate-to-long-term contraception and can return every 11-13 weeks
- Women who do not plan a pregnancy soon after DMPA discontinuation
- Women who want privacy, convenience, and high efficacy
- Women who want or need to avoid estrogen:
  - Women with personal history of thrombosis (WHO: 2) or strong family history of venous thromboembolism (WHO: 1)
  - Recently postpartum women (WHO: 1)
  - Women who are exclusively breast-feeding beyond 6 weeks postpartum (WHO: 1). There is debate about use of DMPA in breastfeeding women less than 6 weeks PP (see p. 120 under INITIATING METHOD POSTPARTUM) ◀
  - Smokers over age 35 (WHO: 1)
  - Women who fear chloasma or had vomiting, migraine headaches, hypertriglyceridemia, or other estrogen-related side effects
- Women who use drugs which affect liver clearance (except aminoglutethimide)
- Women with anemia, fibroids, seizure disorder (WHO 1), sickle cell disease (WHO: 1), endometriosis, hypertriglyceridemia (WHO: 2), systemic lupus erythematosus or coagulation disorder (hyper- or hypo-coagulation)
- Physically compromised women for whom bleeding is a nuisance or a problem ◀

Adolescent women – positive features: (WHO: 2)
- Extremely effective with long carry-over if patient returns late for reinjection (see Figure 27.1, p. 128); Decreases menstrual cramps and pain
- Privacy and confidentiality possible

Adolescent women – special issues:
- For some teens (especially those who have experienced an unintended pregnancy) may be only acceptable method that offers high efficacy
- May be associated with significant weight gain, acne, complexion changes
- Requires periodic reinjections

Bone Mineral Density and Depo-Provera ◀
Women who used DMPA for at least 5 years have significantly reduced bone mineral density (BMD) of lumbar spine and femoral neck, particularly after 15 years of use and if started before age 20 [Cundy-1998]. But effect is almost completely reversible, even after ≥ 4 years of DMPA use, comparable to the effect and reversal seen after lactation [Petitti-2000]. All women placed on DMPA including teens should be encouraged to take calcium tabs and to exercise regularly

PRESCRIBING PRECAUTIONS: Women unwilling to accept a change in their ◀ menstrual periods

- Pregnancy
- Undiagnosed abnormal vaginal bleeding
- Unable to tolerate injections; afraid of shots
- History of breast cancer, MI or stroke
- Blood pressure >160 systolic or > 100 diastolic ◀
- Current venous thromboembolism (unless anticoagulated)
- Active viral hepatitis ◀
- Known hypersensitivity to Depo-Provera

DRUG INTERACTIONS: Aminoglutethimide (Cytodren), used to treat Cushings disease, reduces DMPA efficacy

123

MEDICAL ELIGIBILITY CHECKLIST

Ask the client the questions below. If she answers NO to ALL the questions, then she CAN use DMPA if she wants. If she answers YES to a question below, follow the instructions

1. Do you think you are pregnant?

☐ No ☐ Yes   Assess if pregnant. If she might be pregnant, give her condoms or spermicide to use until reasonably sure that she is not pregnant. Then she can start DMPA

2. Do you plan to become pregnant in the next year?

☐ No ☐ Yes   Use another method with less potential delay in return of fertility

3. Do you have serious medical problems such as heart attack (WHO: 3), severe chest pain, or uncontrolled high blood pressure (WHO: 2 or 3)? Have you ever had such problems? (See page A-3)

☐ No ☐ Yes   In general, do not provide DMPA if she reports heart attack, stroke, heart disease due to blocked arteries, severe high blood pressure (systolic ≥ 160 or diastolic ≥ 100), diabetes for more than 20 years, or damage to vision, kidneys, or nervous system caused by diabetes or by HTN. Help her choose another effective method. All the above conditions receive a "3" in the 2001 WHO Medical Eligibility Criteria (see Appendix pages A-2 and A-3)

4. Do you have or have you recently had breast cancer (WHO: 3 or 4)? (See page A-5)

☐ No ☐ Yes   Do not provide DMPA. Help her choose a method without hormones

5. Do you have jaundice, cirrhosis of the liver, a liver infection or tumor? (Are her eyes or skin unusually yellow?) (See page A-5)

☐ No ☐ Yes   Perform physical exam or refer. If she has serious liver disease (jaundice, painful or enlarged liver, viral hepatitis, liver tumor), do not provide DMPA. Refer for care. Help her choose a method without hormones

6. Do you have vaginal bleeding that is unusual for you? (See page A-4)

☐ No ☐ Yes   If she is not pregnant but has unexplained vaginal bleeding that suggest an underlying medical condition, assess and treat any underlying condition as appropriate, or refer. Provide DMPA based on findings

7. For patients who delivered < than 1 year ago. Did you have diabetes (See p. A-6) with this pregnancy and do you plan to breastfeed (See p. A-2)?

☐ No ☐ Yes   Advise patient there may be some increased risk of developing glucose intolerance or frank diabetes the first year if she has no periods on DMPA. If there is no other good method for her, she may still use Depo-Provera

INITIATING METHOD (see Figure 27.1, page 128)

A pelvic exam is not necessary prior to the initiation of this method

Cycling women:
- Preferred start time is during first 5 days from the start of menses
- Alternative: inject anytime in the cycle when not pregnant, back-up for 7 days

Postpartum women: May give first injection prior to hospital discharge. Special considerations:
- After severe obstetrical blood loss, delay injection until lochia stops
- If woman has history or high risk for severe postpartum depression, observe carefully ◄ and delay injection at least 4-6 weeks
- Breast-feeding women: If mother's nutrition is adequate, may start DMPA immediately. Otherwise, wait 4-6 week.

Women who have spontaneous or therapeutic abortion: May initiate immediately.

Women switching methods:
- May start anytime patient is known not to be pregnant
- If switching from non-hormonal method, offer same options as cycling women

INSTRUCTIONS FOR PATIENT
- **Do NOT massage area where shot was given** (massaging area may reduce duration of action and thereby effectiveness)
- Expect irregular bleeding/spotting in beginning. Usually decreases over time
- Return at any time spotting or bleeding is bothersome. Treatments available that may make bleeding pattern more tolerable
- It is not harmful or dangerous if you do not have periods while you use DMPA
- Weight change is common. Watch what you eat and exercise

WEIGHT GAIN: A TEACHABLE MOMENT

When you see a patient who is very heavy or has gained some weight that disturbs her, you have a teachable moment. BE PREPARED FOR THAT TEACHABLE MOMENT. Here are several suggestions that take but a minute to share.

Helping someone to lose weight in 60 seconds!

1. Eat less (small, frequent meals helps some to lose weight)
2. Exercise more
3. Find patterns of eating and exercising that you enjoy! You won't do them for long unless you enjoy the process.
4. Call Overeaters Anonymous (OA), a free source of love and caring. OA works! www.overeatersanonymous.org
5. Drink 8-10 glasses of water daily

- Be sure to take 1000 mg (women over age 25) to 1300 mg (adolescent women) calcium every day to build your bones. Take calcium tablets like calcium carbonate or TUMS daily if your diet does not include enough calcium. Get weight bearing exercise 3 times a week (good for general health)
- Return in 11-13 weeks for your next injection. Use abstinence after 13 weeks
- Have condoms and EC ready to use if you are ever late coming for your re-injection
- Pregnancy is very rare, but return for care promptly if you develop any pregnancy symptoms
- Serious complications with Depo-Provera are rare, but return if you have worsening severe headaches; heavy bleeding; depression; severe lower abdominal pain; problems at the shot site (pus, pain or bleeding) or if you think you may be pregnant

125

FOLLOW-UP

- Are you experiencing spotting or irregular bleeding? Have you missed periods or had ◄— very light periods? Are you concerned about your pattern of bleeding?
- Did you have pain at the injection site after previous injection?
- Have you felt depressed or had major mood changes?
- Have you gained 5 pounds or more? (See WEIGHT GAIN, A TEACHABLE MOMENT, p. 125) Be sure to weigh patients at each visit. This means at **each and every visit** ◄—
- Do you have any increase in your headaches?
- Have you had the feeling that you may be pregnant?
- Did you have any problems returning on time for this injection?
- Do you plan to have children? OR Do you plan to have more children?
- What are you doing to protect yourself from STIs?

STRUCTURED COUNSELING FOR DEPO-PROVERA PATIENTS WORKS!

- Discontinuation rates for DMPA users at 1 year are high in the absence of structured ◄— counseling: 70% in a New York study of low-income women *[Polaneczky-1996]*; 43.4% in a rural Mexican study *[Canto-DeCetina-2001]*
- Importance of focused, structured, repeated counseling at initiation and follow-up visits can't be overstated. See STRUCTURED COUNSELING p. 14
- Structured counseling may include repetition, having patient repeat back instructions, showing videotapes, providing videotapes, audiotapes and written instructions and asking focused questions such as "What has happened to your pattern of bleeding?", "Have your periods become extremely light?", OR "Does your pattern of bleeding bother you?" rather than unfocused questions like "Are you having any problems?"
- Structured counseling in Mexico lowered DMPA discontinuation from amenorrhea, irregular bleeding and heavy bleeding from 32% to 8%. Discontinuation from amenorrhea fell from 17 to 3%; from SPT or BTB from 10 to 3%; and from heavy bleeding from 5 to 2% *[Canto-DeCetina-2001]* ◄—
- Weight should be taken at each visit and weight control discussed carefully if there has been weight gain (see progressive weight gain p. 122 and WEIGHT GAIN: A TEACHABLE MOMENT p. 125)

PROBLEM MANAGEMENT
Administration problems

Allergic reaction or vasovagal reaction:

In acute setting, provide support as needed. Benadryl may reduce pruritus and swelling. Oxygen and other resuscitation may be needed for severe reactions (extremely rare). Most allergic manifestations subside in 1 week or so. Refer if symptoms severe or do not improve appropriately. Avoid future injections and help her choose a different method

Vaginal dryness (dyspareunia) or atrophic vaginitis:

May be due to hypoestrogenism. Consider measuring E_2 levels and giving physiologic replacement dose of estrogen, if needed. Consider estrogen vaginal cream, ring, tablets or systemic estrogen (tablets or patch) supplementation. Dyspareunia may be relieved with lubricant

Pain or infection at injection site:

Offer anti-inflammatory medications. Rule out infection or needle damage to nerve, etc. Provide appropriate antibiotics if infected. Avoid massaging area for first several hours after injection. It is wise to avoid injections at sites at risk for massage by daily activities

Patient returns early (<11 weeks) wanting reinjection (eg b/c of travel): May give DMPA ◄

Patient returns late (>13 weeks) for reinjection: See Figure 27.1 on page 128

Switching to another method (eg OCs, IUD, etc) from DMPA: Initiate new method at any time convenient for patient. Preferred time would be near end of effectiveness of last DMPA injection unless switching to OCs, patch or vaginal rings to control menstrual disorders on DMPA. Do NOT wait until next menses to start pills. She may have ◄ amenorrhea for a number of months after DMPA

Transitioning perimenopausal women: See Figure 27.2 on page 129

Problems with usage:

Weight gain:
Advise patient to watch her caloric intake carefully and to increase exercise. Discontinue method if weight gain is excessive or unacceptable

Heavy bleeding:
- Rule out pregnancy, cervical infection, and cervical cancer
- Rule out anemia - recommend iron rich foods and/or supplements
- May treat with NSAIDs or low dose estrogen supplements:
  - Ibuprofen 800 mg orally every 8 hours for 3 days
  - Conjugated equine estrogen (0.625, 1.25, or 2.5 mg) orally once a day up to four times per day for 4-6 days OR ethinyl estradiol 20 mcg daily x 21 days
  - Estrogenic COCs for 1-2 months (in addition to DMPA use)

NOTE: Physiologic estrogen replacement may be continued indefinitely with DMPA use. COCs should be limited to next injection or two. NSAIDs may be used periodically with limit of 2400 mg of ibuprofen per 24 hour period. Avoid NSAIDs in patients with GI disorder or asthma

Irregular bleeding and spotting:
- Rule out infection or cervical lesions as source
- Reassure that cumulative blood loss is usually less not more ◄
- Reassure that irregular spotting and bleeding is to be expected in first several months
- May use same therapies as outlined in heavy bleeding section above

Amenorrhea:
- Reassure her that this is not a medical problem. Do pregnancy test if she has other Sx. Switch method if patient desires menses (consider Lunelle, patch, ring, COCs). Even if she switches to another hormonal method or stops DMPA, menses may not return for months

Depression:
- Evaluate suicide potential and refer immediately, if indicated. Patient should avoid alcohol
- Explain that DMPA usually does not worsen depression. Start antidepressant therapy, if needed. Discontinue DMPA if you or your patient has any misgivings about continuing its use

FERTILITY AFTER USE

- Return to baseline fertility is delayed on average but is excellent after using DMPA
- Average of 9-10 months delay to conception after last shot. (Delay not increased with increased duration of use). More than 90% of women become pregnant within 2 years
- Because anovulation may last for more than 1 year, women who know they will want to become pregnant within one year of cessation of use would be wise to consider another option, especially women over 35 years of age ◄
- Women who do not want to await spontaneous return of ovulation will require gonadotrophin therapy to induce ovulation. Gonadotropins will not overcome effect of DMPA on cervical mucus

Figure 27.1 Initial Injection or Late Reinjection (more than 13 weeks since last injection) of DMPA or Switching From DMPA to COCs or Another Hormonal Method*

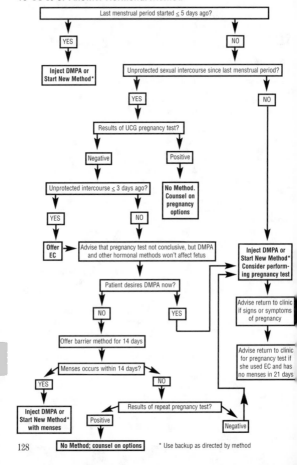

* Use backup as directed by method

Figure 27.2 Making Transition from DMPA to Menopause, With or Without Hormone Replacement Therapy (HRT)

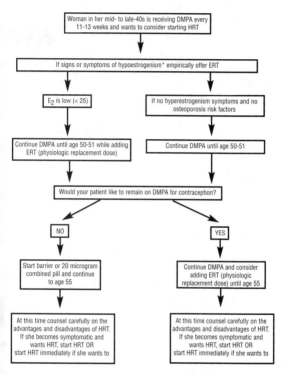

Woman in her mid- to late-40s is receiving DMPA every 11-13 weeks and wants to consider starting HRT

↓

If signs or symptoms of hypoestrogenism* empirically offer ERT

E_2 is low (< 25)

↓

Continue DMPA until age 50-51 while adding ERT (physiologic replacement dose)

If no hyperestrogenism symptoms and no osteoporosis risk factors

↓

Continue DMPA until age 50-51

Would your patient like to remain on DMPA for contraception?

NO

↓

Start barrier or 20 microgram combined pill and continue to age 55

↓

At this time counsel carefully on the advantages and disadvantages of HRT. If she becomes symptomatic and wants HRT, start HRT OR start HRT immediately if she wants to

YES

↓

Continue DMPA and consider adding ERT (physiologic replacement dose) until age 55

↓

At this time counsel carefully on the advantages and disadvantages of HRT. If she becomes symptomatic and wants HRT, start HRT OR start HRT immediately if she wants to

* DMPA can suppress gonadotropins, so measuring FSH or LH is not informative of menopausal state. DMPA use decreases endogenous estrogen levels. Long-term DMPA users in their 40s may benefit from estrogen supplementation. Kaunitz supplements long-term DMPA users in their 40s with 1.25 mg of conjugated estrogen (or equivalent drug). Arbitrarily, at age 55, each woman, if she wants to and understands the risks and benefits, can be switched to conventional HRT. This is easy and minimizes need for laboratory testing, addresses the bone density issue, contraception, and vasomotor concerns while maintaining amenorrhea. [Kaunitz, 1998]

IMPLANTS: IMPLANON - THE SINGLE ETONOGESTREL IMPLANT

DESCRIPTION: Now available in the Netherlands, UK, Sweden, Germany, Belgium, Finland, Switzerland, Denmark and Austria. Coming soon to U.S.

Single implant is 4-cm long and 2 mm in diameter (5 mm longer than one Norplant implant), with a membrane of ethylene vinyl acetate copolymer and with a core of 68 mg of etonogestrel (the new name for 3-ketodesogestrel). Progestin released at rate of 60 μg per day for effective life of 2 years. Implant is placed under the skin of upper arm with a disposable, preloaded inserter

(stamp: NOT AVAILABLE TO WOMEN IN THE US!)

EFFECTIVENESS: Similar to Norplant, with effective life of 3 years. No pregnancies in earliest studies, some reported to FDA since ◄

MECHANISM
- Within 24 hours of insertion thick cervical mucus prevents normal sperm transport
- Inhibition of ovulation (greater than with Norplant implants)(0% in first 2 years)
- Atrophic endometrium: inadequate development of secretory endometrium

COST: Not determined

ADVANTAGES

Menstrual: Decreased menstrual and ovulatory cramping or pain; overall, less bleeding than with Norplant

Sexual/psychological:
- Sexual intercourse may be more pleasurable because fear of pregnancy is reduced
- Applied at time independent of sexual intercourse—allows spontaneity

Cancers/tumors and masses: None

Other:
- High continuation rate in clinical trials. Cyclic headaches may improve
- Single implant is easier and faster to insert and remove than multiple implants and is usually accomplished with only scapel and gently blunt pressure. The copolymer ◄ also may create less scarring and therefore be easier to remove

DISADVANTAGES

Menstrual:
- Irregular menstrual bleeding not uncommon initially
- Amenorrhea in 20% of users with time

Sexual/psychological:
- Irregular bleeding may inhibit sexual intercourse
- Insertion and removal require procedures, for which special training is needed

Cancers/tumors and masses: None

Other:
- No STI protection
- Hormonal side effects: headache is most common

COMPLICATIONS (see Norplant) Removal complications much less frequent

PRESCRIBING PRECAUTIONS, CANDIDATES FOR USE, MEDICAL ELIGIBILITY CHECKLIST, INITIATING METHOD (Next edition when Implanon will possibly be available)

INSTRUCTIONS FOR PATIENT: Irregular bleeding is to be expected. If your pattern of bleeding is unacceptable, come back because there are several treatments that make your bleeding pattern more acceptable. Amenorrhea more likely than with Norplant, but less likely than with DMPA

FOLLOW-UP, PROBLEM MANAGEMENT (details - next edition!)

FERTILITY AFTER USING: Return to baseline fertility is rapid and complete; 94% ovulate within month of removal

IMPLANTS: JADELLE - 2 IMPLANTS

DESCRIPTION:
- Norplant II or Jadelle is very similar to Norplant but consists of 2 slightly larger "rods" rather than 6 "capsules"
- Actually has been approved as a 3-year contraceptive by U.S. FDA. Not yet marketed in U.S.
- 5-year contraceptive effectiveness rates documented (Sivin et al)

DESCRIPTION: 6 soft plastic (silastic) implants (34 mm in length and 2.4 mm in diameter) are inserted into the subcutaneous tissue beneath the skin of the medial aspect of a woman's non-dominant upper arm. Each implant is filled with 36 mg of levonorgestrel powder, which is slowly released through micropores in the implant to achieve an average plasma concentration of 0.30 ng/ml over 5 years. Since Norplant is not currently available, much of the information on this excellent method has been left out of this edition (See the 2000-2001 edition of *Managing Contraception*). As of March 2003, there are no plans for Norplant to be reintroduced ◄ in the U.S. For more information: ***www.popcouncil.org*** or ***www.wyeth.com/news***. The ◄ latest data show that the last Norplant lot is effective. Women no longer have to use backup◄ as was previously recommended (from Wyeth bulletin).

EFFECTIVENESS *[Trussell J IN Contraceptive Technology-2003]*

- Product labeling indicates the system is effective for up to 5 years. Is effective for 7 years or more in women ≤ 154 pounds ◄

Perfect use failure rate in first year: 0.05% (1 woman in 2,000)
Typical use failure rate in first year: 0.05%
Cumulative 7 year failure rate: 1.9% *[Contraception 61:187, 2000]*
(failure rate higher beyond 5 years in obese women (>90 kg or 200 pounds); ◄ recommend back up)

MECHANISMS

The primary mechanism of action is to thicken the cervical mucus consistently throughout the cycle to block sperm penetration into the female upper reproductive tract and avoid fertilization. In the first 1-2 years of use when the circulating levonorgestrel levels are higher, ovulation is blocked in most women. However, by the fifth year of use, nearly 90% of users are routinely ovulating. The progestin may create an inadequate luteal phase and a uterine environment that is suboptimal for implantation, but the clinical significance of these mechanisms has not been demonstrated.

COST: The Contraception Foundation (1-800-760-9030) funds are available to ◄ pay for simple or complicated removals for some uninsured women

ADVANTAGES

Menstrual:
- Decreases cumulative blood loss (mean monthly blood loss 25 cc vs 35 cc in controls)
- Decreases menstrual cramping and pain
- Decreases pain with ovulation in early years (Mittelschmerz)

Sexual/psychological:
- Reduction in pregnancy risk may make sexual activity more pleasurable
- Convenient: no action required at time of intercourse

Cancers, tumors, and masses:
- May reduce risk of endometrial cancer and/or ovarian cancer. No data

Others:

- Highly effective and inexpensive
- Convenient: single insertion provides at least 5 years of protection
- Private: if correctly inserted deeply enough below skin, palpable but usually not obviously visible
- Decreases risk of PID
- Extremely low doses of progestin, no estrogen. Good option for women who can not use estrogen

Adolescent Issues:

- Adolescents have higher continuation rates with Norplant than with COCs or DMPA
- Lower pregnancy rates have been seen in teen mothers using Norplant compared to those using contraceptive pills

DISADVANTAGES
Menstrual:

- Irregular menses is very common during first year
- Usually in first year, women have more days of spotting and bleeding than nonusers, but have less total blood loss
- 20% have amenorrhea or oligomenorrhea
- After 6-12 months, many women re-establish predictable menstrual patterns, but significant minority persists with unpredictable patterns

Sexual/Psychological:

- Spotting and bleeding may interfere with sexual activities
- Possible increase in mood changes, depression, anxiety, irritability, fatigue
- Fear of needles (for injecting local anesthesia) or scalpel may make this an unacceptable choice
- Dislike of foreign bodies or hormones may preclude selection of this method

Cancers, tumors or masses:

- Ovarian enlargement due to less suppression of FSH may lead to persistent ovarian follicles. Most follicular cysts regress spontaneously; watchful waiting is treatment for asymptomatic women

Others:

- Offers no protection against STIs. Must use condoms if at risk
- Insertion and removal require special procedure by trained medical personnel. Patient unable to discontinue method by herself
- Weight changes reported. Over half of women gain weight; about 20% lose weight. However, average 5-year weight gain similar to women not using Norplant
- Other hormonally-related side effects: breast tenderness, headaches, bloating, acne, vaginal discharge, hair growth, scalp hair loss, skin discoloration over implants, etc.
- Insertion/removal related issues: high initial cost, possible infection or scarring, expulsion, nerve or muscle damage (exceedingly rare), bruising and/or pain after procedure.

COMPLICATIONS: *See Managing Contraception 2000-2001*

CANDIDATES FOR USE: *See Managing Contraception 2000-2001*

PRESCRIBING PRECAUTIONS: *See Managing Contraception 2000-2001*

MEDICAL ELIGIBILITY CHECKLIST: *See Managing Contraception 2000-2001*

INITIATING METHOD: *See Managing Contraception 2000-2001*

PRACTICAL TIPS ON PROPER NORPLANT INSERTION:
See Managing Contraception 2000-2001

INSTRUCTIONS FOR PATIENT: *See Managing Contraception 2000-2001*
• If you move and want implants removed, you may call the Norplant Foundation
  for names of clinicians who will remove implants and to get help with finances if needed.
  The number to call is 1-800-760-9030

FOLLOW-UP: *See Managing Contraception 2000-2001*

PROBLEM MANAGEMENT: *See Managing Contraception 2000-2001*

PRACTICAL TIPS ON PROPER NORPLANT REMOVAL
*Learning proper removal techniques requires formal training under direct
supervision. The tips that follow are brief reminders only:*
• Wyeth-Ayerst and Contraception Foundation provide a video on Norplant removal ◄—
  that is essential for clinicians to view prior to first Norplant removals
• Use arm model to practice removal
• Identify both proximal and distal ends of each implant. Mark both ends
• Place anesthesia at the site of incision and beneath the distal one third to one half of each
  implant. Add NaHCO$_3$ to lidocaine to decrease stinging. Initially, inject approximately 3 cc
  of 1% lidocaine (some add 1:100,000 epinephrine). Have an additional 3-5 cc ready to
  provide additional anesthesia if needed.
• Three major techniques have been developed for implant removal. Learn all three to use
  in different situations. In each case, the goal is to isolate each implant in turn, incise
  through its surrounding fibrous sheath and remove only the implant.
  1. *Standard technique:* (see figure 27.3) Horizontal incision at base of implants. Dissect
     beneath tips to create plane. Grasp each implant with curved forceps and bring to
     incision. Incise through the fibrous sheath and grasp the implant with straight clamp
     and remove it (average removal time for 6 capsules is 20 minutes)

**Figure 27.3: Use of hemostat to remove implant while clinician's finger
pushes implant towards incision***

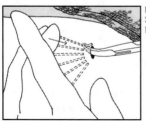

Hatcher RA, et al. *Contraceptive
Technology*. 17th ed. New York: Ardent
Media, 1998.

2. *Instrument-less (fingers-only) technique:* Works well for superficial implants with tips all converging to same point. Infuse area at base with 0.1 cc local anesthesia. Cut directly down to implant and squeeze out through tiny incision. Manipulate subsequent implants out through same incision. (Learning curve is same as Standard technique. Patient satisfaction is very high)

3. *"Norgrasp" or Modified-U technique:* (see figure 27.4) Make vertical incision and create plane laterally beneath implants. Grasp each implant in turn with modified no-scalpel vasectomy clamp (Norgrasp clamp). Incise fibrous sheath and remove implants (Average removal time 6.6 minutes. Quick learning curve)

Figure 27.4: U-technique for Norplant removal*

Hatcher RA, et al *Contraceptive Technology*.
17th ed. New York: Ardent Media, 1998:489

- Show patient all 6 implants
- Close incision with Steri-strips and snug pressure bandage
- Advise patient that she may make dressing looser if she ◄ has swelling or tingling in the affected arm
- Review post procedure instructions with patient (ice, elevation, ibuprofen)

FERTILITY AFTER USE

- Return to baseline fertility is rapid and complete
- Levonorgestrel disappears within 2 days
- Must initiate another method immediately if she does not want to become pregnant

C H A P T E R   2 8

Female Sterilization: Tubal Ligation or Occlusion
www.engenderedhealth.org or www.plannedparenthood.org

DESCRIPTION
Surgery to interrupt the patency of fallopian tubes to prevent pregnancy. In 1995 in the United States, 24% of married women reported having had tubal sterilization while 15% reported that their husbands had had a vasectomy. *[Chandra, 1998]* Approximately half of female sterilizations in the USA are done in the immediate postpartum period within 48 hours of delivery *[Peterson, 1998]*

EFFECTIVENESS
Failure rates differ by sterilization method and patient's age

Table 28.1 Cumulative 10-year failure rates for some methods of voluntary female sterilization methods*

Method	Failure rate (highest rate)	
Post partum salpingectomy	0.8%*	For each sterilization method, at least 50% more failures were ascertained AFTER 2 YEARS as had been identified in the 2 years immediately following the sterilization procedure
Silastic bands	1.8%*	
Interval partial salpingectomy	2.0%*	
Bipolar cautery	2.5%*	
Spring clip	3.7%*	
Filshie clip	0.9%+	

* U.S. Collaborative Review of Sterilization. The risk of pregnancy after tubal sterilization. Am J Obstet Gynecol 1996;174:1161-70.

+ Filshie clip (0.9% failure rate - 7 years) [Chi-Chen Contraception 1987;35:171-8]

- Younger women had higher failure rates
- All methods require proper application to maximize effectiveness
- Teaching institution rates(above study) may differ from private settings

MECHANISM : Interruption of patency of the fallopian tubes thereby preventing fertilization

LAPAROSCOPIC STERILIZATION: TRANSABDOMINAL
Bipolar cautery:
- Apply to area with no vessels ascending through broad ligament, where the diameter of tube similar on either side of damaged area (at least 3 cm from uterotubal junction). Thoroughly cauterize tissue using bipolar cutting current of 25 Watts passes through jaws of instrument. Bipolar cautery has the highest risk of subsequent fistulization and ectopic pregnancy. It replaced previous method of unipolar cautery, which was ◀━━ associated with risk of inadvertent thermal injury

Silastic band: (Fallope ring, Yoon band)
- Apply over knuckle of tube at least 3 cm from utero-tubal junction. Loop of tube should clearly contain two complete ligaments of tube. Good potential for reversibility

Hulka-Clemens clip (spring clip):
- Spring-loaded clip. Apply to isthmic portion of tube. 1-2 cm distal to cornu at an angle of 90% relative to long axis of tube. High potential for reversibility. Highest failure rate

Filshie clip:
- Hinged titanium with cured silicone rubber clip. Apply to isthmic portion of tube, 1 to 2 cm from cornu. High potential for reversibility

Figure 28.1 Laparoscopic Technique Diagrams

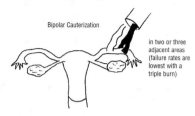

Bipolar Cauterization

in two or three adjacent areas (failure rates are lowest with a triple burn)

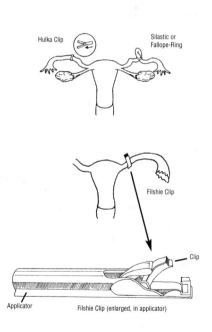

Hulka Clip

Silastic or Fallope-Ring

Filshie Clip

Clip

Applicator

Filshie Clip (enlarged, in applicator)

POSTPARTUM OR INTERVAL MINI-LAPAROTOMY METHODS

Modified Pomeroy:
- Ligation at the base of a loop of isthmic portion of tube with plain catgut suture followed by excision of the knuckle of tube. Good potential for reversal ◄

Modified Parkland:
- Excision of segment of isthmic portion of tube after separate ligation of cut ends

Irving:
- Doubly ligate and sever tube. Bury proximal stump into uterus and put distal stump into mesosalpinx. Poor potential for reversal

Uchida:
- Inject mesenteric part of tube with saline. Divide muscular part of tube/excise 3-5 cm. Bury proximal tube and exteriorize or excise distal tube. Poor potential for reversal ◄

Fimbriectomy:
- Excision of fimbria of tube. Poor potential for reversal ◄

Figure 28.2 Postpartum Techniques

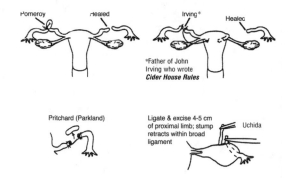

Pomeroy   Healed

Irving*   Healed

*Father of John Irving who wrote *Cider House Rules*

Pritchard (Parkland)

Ligate & excise 4-5 cm of proximal limb; stump retracts within broad ligament   Uchida

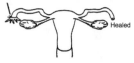

Fimbriectomy

Healed

COST in 1995 [Trussell - 1995; Smith - 1993]

Managed-Care Setting	Public Provider Setting
$2500	$1200

ADVANTAGES

Menstrual: None

Sexual/psychological: Enhanced enjoyment of sex by reducing worry of pregnancy

Cancers, tumors, and masses:
- Decreased risk of ovarian cancer. Women with BRCA 1 mutations who have undergone a tubal ligation have a 60% lower risk of developing invasive ovarian cancer. [Narod-Lancet 357 (9267): 1467-70, 2001]

Other:
- Permanent and highly effective

DISADVANTAGES

Menstrual:
- Data from 9514 women who underwent tubal sterilization by 6 techniques and followed for up to 5 years suggest no "post-tubal ligation syndrome" and no increases in the amount or duration of menstrual bleeding or menstrual pain. [Peterson, 2000]

Sexual/psychological:
- Regret may occur especially with young patients; counsel well (see Fig. 28.5, p. 142) ◄—

Cancers, tumors, and masses: None

Other:
- Requires outpatient surgery (usually with general anesthesia); Expensive in short term
- If failure occurs, higher risk of ectopic pregnancy (10%-65%)
- Not readily reversible and does not prevent spread of HIV and STIs

COMPLICATIONS [Peterson, 1997]

	Minilaparotomy	Laparoscopy
Minor	11.6%	6.0%
Major	1.5%	0.9%

- Minor complications include infection, wound separation
- Major complications include conversion to laparotomy, hemorrhage, viscus injury especially with cautery, anesthetic complications ◄—
- Major vessel injury risk w/ laparoscopy 3-9/10,000 procedures
- Mortality: 1-2/100,000 procedures (leading cause is general anesthesia)

LONG-TERM RISKS

- Statistically higher risk for subsequent hysterectomy, but only in women who had gynecologic complaints prior to sterilization
- Regret (0.9% - 26.0%) Risk factors include: age under 30, low parity, change in marital status, poverty, minority status, misinformation about permanence or risks, decision made in a hurry. The risk of regret is 40% at 14 years in women having tubal sterilization under 30. **This issue requires careful counseling**

CANDIDATES FOR USE

- Woman who is certain she wants no more children
- Woman over age 21 (only required for Medicaid reimbursement, not for medical requirements)
- Woman with a medical condition that makes pregnancy or use of other contraceptives dangerous
- Woman for whom surgery is considered safe

Adolescents: Not a preferred method, generally higher regret and higher failure rates

ESSURE: TRANSCERVICAL STERILIZATION VIA POLYESTHER FIBERS

www.essure.com Essure is a new approach to transcervical sterilization that causes tubal blockage by encouraging local tissue growth with polyester (PET) fibers *[Valle Fertil Steril 2001]*. An attached outer coiled spring is released that molds to the shape of the interstitial (uterine) portion of each fallopian tube. The device costs $950. *[Ballagh, 2003]*

APPROVED BY FDA NOVEMBER 2002

Figure 28.3 Essure System Overview: Micro-Insert Design

Fibers (PET)
Dynamic Expanding Superelastic Outer Coil
Wound Down Diameter 0.8 mm
Expanded Diameter 1.5 - 2.0 mm
Micro-insert Length = 4cm

Source: Association of Reproductive Health Professionals Trancervical methods in the U.S. pipeline. *Clinical Proceedings* 2002; May:9.

ADVANTAGES

- Provides tubal sterilization in physician's or ambulatory surgery office (average operating time: 13 minutes)
- It is the woman's own tissue plus the implant that causes tubal occlusion
- No major change in a woman's menstrual cycles
- No failures among 453 women relying on Essure for one year following confirmation of tubal blockage at 3 months by hysteroscopy
- There is no need for conscious sedation or general anesthesia (nonsteriodal premedication is strongly recommended to prevent tubal spasm)
- In Pivitol Trial, (Australia, Europe, and the U.S.) 92% of women returned to work in one day, most resumed normal activities the same day as the procedure
- More than 95% of women would recommend procedure to a friend

DISADVANTAGES

- Procedure designed for interval sterilization. It is not to be used at Cesarean section or immediately postpartum *[Bullagh, 2003]*
- Luteal pregnancies occured in 4 of 466 women in spite of negative urine pregnancy tests on the day of the procedure
- It may not be possible to visualize both tubal ostia (this occurs about 2% of the time)
- May require more than one operative procedure
- In only 446 of 518 women (86.1%) could devices be introduced into both tubes at the time of the first procedure
- Tubal spasm may occur
- Expulsion of one or both devices (14 of 466 successful procedure or 3.0%)
- Perforation of the uterus occured during 4 of 466 procedures
- **Hysterosaplingogram done at 3 months to confirm blockage. Until that time couple must use another contraceptive. This functional test to determine if the Essure technique has worked, an HSG, is far more complicated and expensive than the functional test to determine if a vasectomy has worked. This is an important disadvantage of the Essure technique**
- Procedures to reverse this form of sterilization require tubal reimplantation into the uterus and have a much lower success rate and expose a woman to the risk of tubal rupture during a subsequent pregnancy

PRESTERILIZATION COUNSELING CHECKLIST*

- Discuss vasectomy as an alternative
- Insure patient commitment to having no future children, even if something happened to her current family
- Discuss alternative reversible methods and quote their effectiveness. (IUDs are more effective than some forms of tubal sterilization)
- Describe details of surgery (informed consent later) and possible intraoperative and long-term complications (risk for ectopic pregnancy)
- Stress that procedure must be considered irreversible and that about 10% of women regret their decision and answer all of her questions
- Obtain informed consent - No requirement that spouse must be involved

*Adapted from ACOG Technical Bulletin, April 1996.

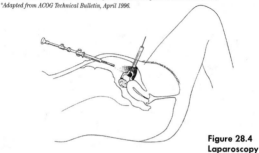

**Figure 28.4
Laparoscopy**

INITIATING METHOD

- Obtain informed consent. Preferable to involve partner in process, but not necessary
- Any time in cycle with certainty of no conception, otherwise follicular timing preferred
- The routine provision of antibiotics is generally NOT recommended *[see ACOG Practice Bulletin No. 23, January, 2001]*

FOLLOW-UP

- Follow up in two weeks for post op wound check. Routine annual gynecology exams

MANAGEMENT OF PROBLEMS

- Anesthesia complications, wound infections, intraperitoneal adhesion formation, hydrosalpinx – managed with standard tools
- Although some women report irregular menses or dysmenorrhea after tubal sterilization, several studies have demonstrated that the syndrome of irregular menses or dysmenorrhea following tubal sterilization does NOT exist *[Peterson-2000]*

FERTILITY AFTER USE

- Women must desire to be permanently sterile because reversal is costly and failure rates are high. In vitro fertilization may be preferable, but many cannot afford this procedure

Figure 28.5 Sterilization Requested by Young Woman

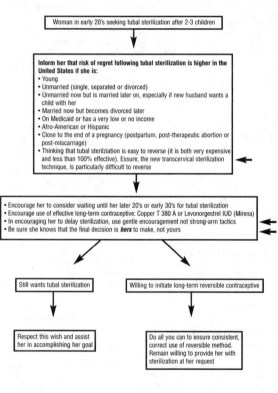

Woman in early 20's seeking tubal sterilization after 2-3 children

Inform her that risk of regret following tubal sterilization is higher in the United States if she is:
- Young
- Unmarried (single, separated or divorced)
- Unmarried now but is married later on, especially if new husband wants a child with her
- Married now but becomes divorced later
- On Medicaid or has a very low or no income
- Afro-American or Hispanic
- Close to the end of a pregnancy (postpartum, post-therapeutic abortion or post-miscarriage)
- Thinking that tubal sterilization is easy to reverse (it is both very expensive and less than 100% effective). Essure, the new transcervical sterilization technique, is particularly difficult to reverse

- Encourage her to consider waiting until her later 20's or early 30's for tubal sterilization
- Encourage use of effective long-term contraceptive: Copper T 380 A or Levonorgestrel IUD (Mirena)
- In encouraging her to delay sterilization, use gentle encouragement not strong-arm tactics
- Be sure she knows that the final decision is *hers* to make, not yours

Still wants tubal sterilization

Willing to initiate long-term reversible contraceptive

Respect this wish and assist her in accomplishing her goal

Do all you can to ensure consistent, correct use of reversible method. Remain willing to provide her with sterilization at her request

CHAPTER 29

Male Sterilization: Vasectomy
www.engenderedhealth.org or www.plannedparenthood.org

DESCRIPTION
Permanent male contraception. Outpatient surgical procedure. No-scalpel technique punctures scrotum, delivers vas; ligates or cauterizes vas

EFFECTIVENESS (See Table 13.2, p. 38)
Perfect use failure rate in first year: 0.10%
Typical use failure rate in first year: 0.15%
[Trussell J, IN Contraceptive Technology, 2004]

Although vasectomy is safer and potentially more effective than tubal sterilization, as of mid-2000, there are only 4 nations in the world where vasectomies exceed tubal sterilizations: Great Britain, the Netherlands, New Zealand and Bhutan.

MECHANISM
Interrupts vas deferens preventing passage of sperm into seminal fluid and female reproductive tract

vas deferens isolated following incision with scalpel

ADVANTAGES
Menstrual: None
Sexual/psychological:
- Sexual intercourse may be more enjoyable because fear of pregnancy decreased
- Permits man opportunity to take on an important contraceptive role
- No interference during sexual intercourse and no contraceptive burden for female
Cancers, tumors, and masses: None
Other:
- Simpler, safer and more effective than female sterilization
- Cost-effective
- Convenient
- Shares contraception responsibility with partner
- No supplies or further clinic visits needed after sperm count has been documented to be zero
- General anesthesia rarely required

DISADVANTAGES
Menstrual: None
Sexual/ psychological:
- Some men resist vasectomy fearing that it will interfere with sexual function (it doesn't) and because they feel contraception is solely the woman's responsibility (it isn't)
- Regret at a later time possible
- Will need back-up method until sperm count reaches zero. Female partner may still need contraception if she has other partners or if STI protection needed
Cancers, tumors, and masses: None
Other:
- Does not reduce risk for STIs; will still need to use condom if at risk
- Short-term post-operative discomfort, bruising, and swelling
- Requires surgical procedure by trained provider

COMPLICATIONS
- Surgically related complaints such as hematoma, bruising, wound infection, or adverse reaction to local anesthesia
- Severe chronic pain (2%) *[Choe, Kirkema - 1996]* ◄
- Later regret possible

143

CANDIDATES FOR USE
Male who: Desires a permanent, effective method of contraception
Adolescents: Not a preferred method

INITIATING METHOD
- Take preoperative history; make general health assessment
- Obtain informed consent. In general, try to involve partner
- Carefully counsel, especially about permanence of method
- Advise patient to bathe genital area and upper thighs prior to surgery; wear clean, loose-fitting clothes to facility; take no medication 24 hours before procedure

PRESCRIBING PRECAUTIONS
- Current infection of penis, prostate, or scrotum
- Current skin infection over incision site
- Fear of needles or scalpels (scalpels not required if no-scalpel vasectomy)

INSTRUCTIONS FOR PATIENT
- Apply ice pack to incision site to decrease swelling, pain and bruising. Small packages of frozen peas conform well around the scrotum
- Keep area dry for two days – wear snug underwear and pants to provide support where needed
- If any symptoms or signs of infection develop, seek help immediately.
- Return as directed for sperm counts. Use other forms of contraception until two consecutive sperm samples show no sperm (a zero sperm count)

FOLLOW-UP
- Have you had your semen tested for the presence of sperm? If yes, were sperm absent?

PROBLEM MANAGEMENT
Wound infection: Treat with antibiotics. Drain and treat any abscesses
Hematoma: Apply warm moist packs to scrotum. Provide scrotal support
Granuloma: Observe; usually it will resolve itself
Pain at site: If no infection, provide scrotal support and analgesics
Excessive swelling: If large and painful, may require surgery. Provide scrotal support if hematoma
Chronic persistent pain considered to be severe: [2% - Choe, Kirkema - 1996]. IPPF ◄
Handbook states that this pain can often be relieved by vasovasectomy or decompression of the distended vas deferens releasing the sperm into the scrotal cavity *[Evans, Huezo IPPF Handbook - 1997]*

FERTILITY AFTER USE
- Man must accept that vasectomy is irreversible and permanent
- Microsurgical techniques of reversal now result in return of sperm to ejaculate in over 90% of men, but in pregnancy rates of only 50% or above. Reversibility rates decrease as ◄ time since procedure increases
- Important factors for reversal are
  - skill of microsurgeon
  - length of time from vasectomy
  - presence of antisperm antibodies (man)
  - partner's fertility
  - manner in which vasectomy was performed (amount of vas removed or cauterized)

Figure 29.1 Vasectomy - No-Scapel Techniques

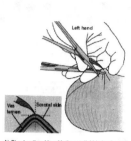

A) Piercing the skin with the medial blade of the dissecting forceps

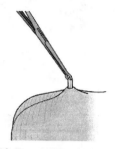

B) Grasping a partial thickness of the elevated vas at the crest of the loop, with only the ringed clamp attached

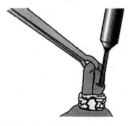

C) Cautery with a blunt wire inserted into the hemitransected vas (done in each direction)

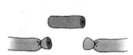

D) Ligation and section

Cornell No-Scalpel Vasectomy Center. No-Scalpel Vasectomy. http://www.vasectomy.com/no-scalpel-vasectomy-diagram.html.2/6/02.

CHAPTER 30

Future Methods
www.popcouncil.org or www.conrad.org OR
www.plannedparenthood.org/ARTICLES/bcfuture-w.html

NEW HORMONAL FORMULATIONS FOR ORAL USE

Several lower-dose COCs are currently available in Europe with EE levels of 10-15 µg

Table 30.1 PROGESTIN-ONLY IMPLANTS

NAME	# CAPSULES	HORMONE	LENGTH OF USE	BIODEGRADABLE
Norplant 2	2	Levonorgestrel	5 yrs.	no
Uniplant	1	nomegestrol		
Nestorone	1	nestorone	2 yrs.	
Implanon	1	etonogestrel	2 yrs.	no	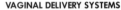
Annuelle	pellets	norethindrone		

VAGINAL DELIVERY SYSTEMS

• Progestin-only vaginal rings: may be worn continuously
   NOTE: Contraceptive vaginal rings that release only a progestin have been studied. Like other progestin-only methods, however, they have a slightly lower effectiveness and slightly higher rates of spotting and bleeding between menses. Progestin-only rings may prove in the future to be a good option for women who are postpartum or breastfeeding or who have contraindications to estrogen containing methods.
• Progesterone daily suppositories

INTRAUTERINE DEVICES

• Gynefix Copper IUD: 6 sleeves of copper on a string that has one end embedded in fundus and other end protruding through cervix for monthly monitoring. IUD has low expulsion rate and cumulative 3-year failure rate of 0.5%
• Fibroplant: progestin-releasing fiber that is fixed in uterine wall

FEMALE BARRIERS

• New prototypes of female condoms
• Femcap: silicone rubber cervical cap; 3 sizes
• Trials beginning on diaphragms that can be fitted by the woman instead of by her clinician
• Protectaid: new vaginal sponges
• Microbicides which are also spermicidal—may not be available for 5-10 years

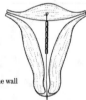

**Figure 30.2
Gynefix
intrauterine
copper IUD**

MALE METHODS

- Male hormonal methods under development often use exogenous progestin or gonadotropin-releasing hormone (GnRH) antagonist to suppress FSH and LH, thereby decreasing spermatogenesis. Replacement testosterone provided
  injectables: progestin + testosterone / GnRH + testosterone
  implants: 2 implant system with GnRH + androgen
- Testosterone (injectable, patch or implant) combined with slow release progestin implant
- Immunocontraception: Methods based on interference of the reproductive process by products of an immune reaction
- "Temporary sterilization"— injecting the vas deferens with a polymer to block sperm
- Anti-sperm compounds, e.g., gossypol from cottonseed oil and Triptolide

NEW EC METHODS: A variety will arise in the future

VACCINES: In phase 1 trials

QUINACRINE STERILIZATION: remains controversial. If 7 quinacrine pellets (252 mg) are introduced into the top of the fundus through an inserter (very much like the inserter used for IUD insertion) and this application is repeated in one month (the Hieu technique) two-year failure rates of 0 *[Sarin-1999]*, 1.2% *[Soroodi-Maghaddam-1996]* have been reported. Other reports have found a pregnancy rate of over 13%. Complications have included anaphylactic shock (2 out of over 130,000), bleeding and rare perforations

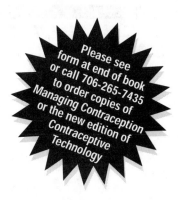

Please see form at end of book or call 706-265-7435 to order copies of Managing Contraception or the new edition of Contraceptive Technology

CHAPTER 31

Sexually Transmissible Infections (STIs)
➤ 2002 CDC Guidelines for Treatment

Complete guidelines at www.cdc.gov/nchstp/od/nchstp.html
www.hab.hrsa.gov   www.aidsinfo.nih.gov ◄

Since women and men seeking contraceptives are also at risk for STIs, we have included in this book information on the treatment of many of the most important STIs. The 2002 guidelines had not yet been formally published by the time *Managing Contraception* went to press. Some of the most important changes in the 2002 CDC Guidelines have been incorporated into the pages that follow.

CLINICAL PREVENTION GUIDELINES

- This section is a summary of selected paragraphs and treatments from the *2002 Guidelines for Sexually Transmitted Diseases* published by the CDC *[CDC, 2002]*
- The specific recommendations presented here are from that document
- Both partners should get tested for STIs, including HIV, before initiating sexual intercourse
- A new condom should be used for each act of insertive intercourse (oral, vaginal or anal)

Prevention Methods
- *Male Condoms*
  - Used consistently and correctly, latex condoms are effective in preventing the transmission of HIV infection and can reduce the risk for other STIs
  - Failure usually results from inconsistent or incorrect use, rather than condom breakage

- *Female Condoms*
  - Laboratory studies indicate that the female condom (Reality) is an effective mechanical barrier to viruses, including HIV
  - Used consistently and correctly, the female condom may substantially reduce risk for STIs including HIV

- *Condoms and Spermicides*
  - Whether condoms used with vaginal application of spermicide are more effective than condoms used without vaginal spermicides has not been determined
  - Therefore, the consistent use of condoms, with or without spermicidal lubricant or vaginal application of spermicide, is recommended

- However, vaginal spermicides containing N-9 are not effective in preventing cervical gonorrhea, chlamydia or HIV infection
- Diaphragm use has been demonstrated to provide some protection against cervical gonorrhea, chlamydia, and trichomoniasis (case control, cross sectional studies)
- Vaginal sponges or diaphragms should not be relied upon to protect women against HIV infection

- *Nonbarrier Contraception, Surgical Sterilization, and Hysterectomy*
  - Hormonal contraception (e.g., oral contraceptives, Norplant, and Depo-Provera) offer no protection against HIV or other STDs
  - Women who use hormonal or intrauterine contraception, have been surgically sterilized, or have had hysterectomies should still be counseled on the use of condoms for HIV/STI protection

SPECIAL POPULATIONS

Pregnant Women
- *Recommended Screening Tests*
  - Syphilis: all pregnant women at first prenatal visit; high risk (high areas of syphilis morbidity) retested in early third trimester and at delivery
  - Hepatitis B surface antigen (HbsAg): all pregnant women first visit
  - *Neisseria gonorrhoeae:* first visit for women at risk or living in an area of high prevalence
  - *Chlamydia trachomatis:* at first prenatal visit and in the third trimester for women at increased risk (i.e., women aged <25 years and women who have a new or more than one sex partner or whose partner has other partners)
  - HIV screening test: encouraged for all pregnant women as routine prenatal test at ◀— the first prenatal visit
  - Bacterial vaginosis (BV): may be performed at the first prenatal visit for patients at high risk for preterm labor (history of prematurity). Current evidence does not support universal testing for BV
  - Papanicolaou (Pap) smear: first visit if no Pap smear has been documented during the preceding year
  - Hepatitis C antibodies should be performed at the first prenatal visit for women at high risk (intravenous drug users, blood transfusions, organ transplant)

- *Other Concerns (Other STI-related Concerns are to Be Considered as Follows:)*
  - Pregnant women who have either primary genital herpes infection, HBV, primary cytomegalovirus (CMV) infection, or Group B streptococcal infection and women who have syphilis and who are allergic to penicillin may need to be referred to an expert for management
  - HbsAg-positive pregnant women should be reported to the local and/or state health department; household and sexual contacts of HbsAg-positive women should be tested and immunized if negative
  - In the absence of lesions during the third trimester, routine serial culture for herpes simplex virus (HSV) is not indicated for women who have a history of recurrent genital herpes. However, obtaining cultures from such women at the time of delivery may be useful in guiding neonatal management. Prophylactic cesarean section is not indicated for women who do not have active genital lesions at the time of delivery
  - The presence of genital warts is not an indication for cesarean section unless size obstructs delivery in labor (rare)

Adolescents
- With limited exceptions, all U.S. adolescents can consent to the confidential diagnosis and treatment of STIs. See Table 6.1, p. 19
- Medical care for STIs can be provided to adolescents without parental consent or knowledge
- Providers should appreciate how important confidentiality is to adolescents

DISEASES CHARACTERIZED BY GENITAL ULCERS

Management of Patients Who Have Genital Ulcers

- In the United States, most young, sexually active patients who have genital ulcers have genital herpes, a smaller percentage have syphilis, or chancroid. Each disease has been associated with an increased risk for HIV infection
- The evaluation of all patients who have genital ulcers should include a serologic test for syphilis and diagnostic evaluation for herpes; in settings where chancroid is prevalent a test for *Haemophilis ducreyi* should be performed. Specific tests (to be used with clinical assessment) for the evaluation of genital ulcers include the following:
  - Serology, dark-field examination or direct immunofluorescence test for *Treponema pallidum*
  - Culture or antigen test for HSV and
  - Culture for *Haemophilus ducreyi*
- HIV testing should be a) performed in the management of patients who have genital ulcers caused by *T. pallidum* or *H. ducreyi* and b) considered for those who have ulcers caused by HSV

CHANCROID (SHAN-kroyd)

Organism: H. ducreyi

Diagnosis: Culture on special medium of *H. ducreyi*, or if the following criteria are met: a) patient has 1 or more ulcers; b) no evidence of syphilis on lab exam after at least 7 days; c) the clinical picture is typical of chancroid and d) test for HSV is negative.

Treatment: Recommended Regimens

Azithromycin	1 g orally in a single dose, OR
Ceftriaxone	250 mg intramuscularly (IM) in a single dose, OR ◄
Ciprofloxacin	500 mg orally twice a day for 3 days, OR
Erythromycin base	500 mg orally three times a day for 7 days.

Follow-up: Re-examine in 3-7 days. If no improvement consider whether a) the diagnosis is correct, b) the patient is coinfected with another STI, c) the patient is infected with HIV, d) the treatment was not taken as instructed, or e) the *H. ducreyi* strain causing the infection is resistant to the prescribed antimicrobial.

- *The time required for complete healing:*
  - Depends on the size of the ulcer; large ulcers may require >2 weeks
  - Healing is slower for some uncircumcised men who have ulcers under the foreskin
  - Resolution of fluctuant lymphadenopathy is slower than that of ulcers and may require drainage, even during otherwise successful therapy
  - Although needle aspiration of buboes is a simple procedure, incision and drainage of buboes may be preferred because of less need for subsequent drainage procedures

Management of Sex Partners: Should be examined and treated regardless of symptoms if they had sexual contact within 10 days of the onset of symptoms

Special Considerations: Pregnancy. The safety of azithromycin for pregnant and lactating women has not been established. Ciprofloxacin is contraindicated during pregnancy. No adverse effects of chancroid on pregnancy outcome or on the fetus have been reported.

GENITAL HERPES SIMPLEX VIRAL (HSV) INFECTION (Her-pes)

Most persons shed the virus intermittently and are unaware that they are infected and are asymptomatic at the time of transmission.

Organisms: HSV-1 and HSV-2

Diagnosis: See complete *2002 CDC Guidelines* or *Contraceptive Technology (18th Edition)*

Counseling: Counseling of these patients should include the following:
- Patients should be advised to abstain from sexual activity when lesions or prodromal symptoms are present and encouraged to inform their sex partners that they have genital herpes
- Latex condoms, when used consistently and correctly, can reduce the risk for genital herpes, when the infected areas are covered or protected by the condom
- Sexual transmission of HSV can occur during asymptomatic periods
- The risk for neonatal infection should be explained to all patients, including men. Childbearing-aged women who have genital herpes should be advised to inform health-care providers who care for them during pregnancy about the HSV infection
- Patients having a first episode of genital herpes should be advised that a) episodic antiviral therapy during recurrent episodes might shorten the duration of lesions and b) suppressive antiviral therapy can ameliorate or prevent recurrent outbreaks

Treatment: 5% to 30% of first-episode cases of genital herpes are caused by HSV-1, but clinical recurrences are much less frequent for HSV-1 than HSV-2 genital infection

---

• HSV, Recommended Regimens for First Clinical Infection

Acyclovir.................................400 mg orally three times a day for 7-10 days, OR
Acyclovir.................................200 mg orally five times a day for 7-10 days, OR
Famciclovir.............................250 mg orally three times a day for 7-10 days, OR
Valacyclovir............................1.0 g orally twice a day for 7-10 days

• HSV, Recommended Regimens for Episodic Recurrent Infection

Acyclovir.................................400 mg orally three times a day for 5 days, OR
Acyclovir.................................200 mg orally five times a day for 5 days, OR
Acyclovir.................................800 mg orally twice a day for 5 days, OR
Famciclovir.............................125 mg orally twice a day for 5 days, OR
Valacyclovir............................500 mg orally twice a day for 3-5 days, OR
Valacyclovir............................1.0 g orally once a day for 5 days

• HSV, Recommended Regimens for Daily Suppressive Therapy

Acyclovir.................................400 mg orally twice a day, OR
Famciclovir.............................250 mg orally twice a day, OR
Valacyclovir............................250 mg orally twice a day, OR
Valacyclovir............................500 mg orally once a day

---

- Valacyclovir 500 mg once a day appears less effective than other valacyclovir dosing regimens in patients who have very frequent recurrences (i.e., >10 episodes per year)
- Valacyclovir and famciclovir appear to be comparable to acyclovir in clinical outcome
- However, valacyclovir and famciclovir may be easier to take

Severe Disease: IV therapy should be provided for patients who have severe disease or complications necessitating hospitalization, such as disseminated infection, pneumonitis, hepatitis, or complications of the central nervous system (e.g., meningitis or encephalitis)

• HSV, Recommended Regimen for Persons with Severe Disease

Acyclovir.................................5-10 mg/kg body weight IV every 8 hours for 5-7 days until clinical resolution is attained

---

Special Considerations:
- *Pregnancy*
  - Available data do not indicate an increased risk for major birth defects in women treated with acyclovir in the first trimester
  - The safety of valacyclovir, and famciclovir therapy in pregnant women has not been established

- *Perinatal Infection*
  - The risk for transmission to the neonate from an infected mother is high (30% - 50%) among women who acquire genital herpes near the time of delivery and is low (3%) among women who have a history of recurrent herpes at term and women who acquire genital HSV during the first half of pregnancy
  - Therefore, prevention of neonatal herpes should emphasize prevention of acquisition of genital HSV infection during late pregnancy
  - Susceptible women whose partners have oral or genital HSV infection, or those whose sex partners' infection status is unknown, should be counseled to avoid unprotected genital and oral sexual contact during late pregnancy
  - The results of viral cultures during pregnancy do not predict viral shedding at the time of delivery, and such cultures are not indicated routinely
  - At the onset of labor, all women should be examined and carefully questioned about whether they have symptoms of HSV. Infants of women who do not have symptoms or signs of HSV infection or its prodrome may be delivered vaginally
  - Cesarean delivery does not completely eliminate the risk for HSV infection in the neonate

GRANULOMA INGUINALE (DONOVANOSIS) (gran-u-LO-ma in-gwi-NAL-e, don-o-van-O-sis)

Organism: *Calymmatobacterium granulomatis* is an intracellular, gram-negative bacterium. It is seen rarely in the USA. Presents as a painless, progressive, vascular, ulcerative lesion with regional lymphadenopathy

Diagnosis: Visualization of Donovan bodies from tissue of lesion

Treatment: Appears to halt progressive destruction of tissue. Prolonged duration of therapy often required to enable granulation and re-epithelialization of the ulcers. Therapy should be continued until all lesions have healed completely

- *Granuloma Inguinale, Recommended Regimens*

Doxycycline............................100 mg orally twice a day for a minimum or 3 weeks

Trimethoprim-
sulfamethoxazole....................One double-strength tablet orally twice a day for a minimum of 3 weeks, OR

- *Granuloma Inguinale, Alternative Regimens*

Ciprofloxacin...........................750 mg orally twice a day for a minimum of 3 weeks, OR

Erythromycin base.................500 mg orally four times a day for a minimum of 3 weeks (for use during pregnancy), OR

Azithromycin...........................1 g orally per week for at least 3 weeks

NOTE: For any of the above regimens, the addition of an aminoglycoside (gentamicin 1 mg/kg IV every 8 hours) should be considered if lesions do not respond within the first few days of therapy

LYMPHOGRANULOMA VENEREUM (LGV) (lim-fo-gran-u-LO-ma ve-nar-E-um)

This is a rare disease in the USA, most frequently manifested in heterosexual men as unilateral tender inguinal nodes and in women and homosexual men with proctocolitis, or inflammatory involvement or perirectal or perianal fistulas or strictures

Organism: Invasive strains L1, L2, or L3 of *Chlamydia trachomatis*

Diagnosis: Serological and exclusion of other ulcerative lesions or those with lymphadenopathy.

Treatment: Treatment cures infection and prevents ongoing tissue damage, although tissue reaction can result in scarring. Buboes may require aspiration through intact skin or incision and drainage to prevent the formation of inguinal/femoral ulcerations.

- *LGV, Recommended Regimen*
  Doxycycline............................100 mg orally twice a day for 21 days OR
- *Alternative Regimen*
  Erythromycin base..................500 mg orally four times a day for 21 days

SYPHILIS   (SIF-i-lis)

Organism: Treponema pallidum (tre-po-NE-ma PAL-e-dum)
Diagnosis: See most recent CDC Guidelines or *Contraceptive Technology*
Treatment:
- Parenteral penicillin G is preferred drug for treatment of all stages of syphilis. The preparation(s) used (i.e., benzathine, aqueous procaine, or aqueous crystalline), the dosage, and the length of treatment depend on the stage and clinical manifestations of disease
- Parenteral penicillin G is the only therapy with documented efficacy for neurosyphilis or for syphilis during pregnancy. Patients who report a penicillin allergy, including pregnant women with syphilis in any stage and patients with neurosyphilis, should be desensitized and treated with penicillin
- The Jarisch-Herxheimer reaction is an acute febrile reaction often accompanied by headache, myalgia, and other symptoms that might occur within the first 24 hours after any therapy for syphilis; patients should be advised of this possible adverse reaction

PRIMARY AND SECONDARY SYPHILIS:

- *Recommended Regimen for Adults*
  Benzathine penicillin G....... 2.4 million units IM in a single dose

Other Management Considerations: All patients who have syphilis should be tested for HIV infection. In geographic areas in which the prevalence of HIV is high, patients who have primary syphilis should be retested for HIV after 3 months if the first HIV test result was negative

Follow-up: Serologic test titers may decline more slowly for patients who previously had syphilis. Patients should be reexamined clinically and serologically at both 6 months and 12 months; also see complete *2002 CDC Guidelines* for more detail

Management of Sex Partners: Sexual transmission of T. pallidum *has occurred only when mucocutaneous syphilitic lesions are present;* such manifestations are uncommon after the first year of infection. However, persons exposed sexually to a patient who has syphilis in any stage should be evaluated clinically and, according to CDC, serologically

Special Considerations
- *Penicillin Allergy:* Nonpregnant penicillin-allergic patients who have primary or secondary syphilis should be treated with one of the following regimens. Close follow-up of such patients is essential. Limited clinical studies suggest that ceftrioxone may be effective for early syphilis. The optional dose and duration of therapy have not been defined, however, some specialists recommend 1 gm daily IM or IV for 8-10 days

- *Recommended Regimens*
  Doxycycline............................100 mg orally twice a day for 2 weeks, OR
  Tetracycline............................500 mg orally four times a day for 2 weeks
- Pregnant patients who are allergic to penicillin should be desensitized, if necessary, and treated with penicillin.

See most recent CDC Guidelines or *Contraceptive Technology*
See most recent CDC Guidelines or *Contraceptive Technology*

DISEASES CHARACTERIZED BY URETHRITIS AND CERVICITIS

Management of Patients Who Have Nongonococcal Urethritis

Diagnosis: Testing for chlamydia is strongly recommended because of the increased utility and availability of highly sensitive and specific testing methods and because a specific diagnosis might improve compliance and partner notification

Treatment:

- *Nongonococcal Urethritis, Recommended Regimens*

Azithromycin...........................1 g orally in a single dose, OR
Doxycycline...........................100 mg orally twice a day for 7 days

- *Nongonococcal Urethritis, Alternative Regimens*

Erythromycin base....................500 mg orally four times a day for 7 days, OR
Erythromycin ethylsuccinate....800 mg orally four times a day for 7 days, OR
Ofloxacin....................300 mg twice a day for 7 days, OR
Levofloxacin.............................500 mg orally once daily for 7 days

Follow-up: If symptoms persist, patients should be instructed to return for reevaluation and to abstain from sexual intercourse even if they have completed the prescribed therapy

Partner Referral: Patients should refer all sex partners within the preceding 60 days for evaluation and treatment

- *Recurrent/Persistent Urethritis, Recommended Treatment*

Metronidazole..........................2 g orally in a single dose, PLUS
Erythromycin base....................500 mg orally four times a day for 7 days, OR
Erythromycin ethylsuccinate....800 mg orally four times a day for 7 days

CHLAMYDIAL INFECTION IN ADOLESCENTS AND ADULTS

Several important sequelae can result from *Chlamydia trachomatis* (kla-MID-e-a tra-KO-ma-tis) infection in women; the most serious of these include PID, ectopic pregnancy, and infertility. Some women who have apparently uncomplicated cervical infection already have subclinical upper reproductive tract infection

Diagnosis: See complete *2002 CDC Guidelines* or *Contraceptive Technology*

Treatment:

- Treatment of infected patients prevents transmission to sex partners and, for infected pregnant women, might prevent transmission to infants during birth
- Treatment of sex partners helps to prevent reinfection of the index patient and infection of other partners
- Coinfection with *C. trachomatis* often occurs among patients who have gonococcal infection; therefore, presumptive treatment of such patients for chlamydia is appropriate (see GONOCOCCAL INFECTION, Dual Therapy for Gonococcal and Chlamydial Infection, p 155)
- The following recommended treatment regimens and the alternative regimens cure infection and usually relieve symptoms:

- *Chlamydia Infection, Recommended Regimens*

Azithromycin.............................1 g orally in a single dose, OR (equally effective) ◄──

Doxycycline...............................100 mg orally twice a day for 7 days

- *Chlamydia Infection, Alternative Regimens*

Erythromycin base....................500 mg orally four times a day for 7 days, OR

Erythromycin ethylsuccinate...800 mg orally four times a day for 7 days, OR

Ofloxacin..................................300 mg orally twice a day for 7 days, OR

Levofloxacin.............................500 mg orally for 7 days

Follow-up: Patients do not need to be retested for chlamydia after completing treatment with doxycycline or azithromycin unless symptoms persist or reinfection is suspected because these therapies are highly efficacious. Consider rescreening for chlamydia infection 3-4 months after treatment due to high prevalence of reinfection, especially for adolescents

Management of Sex Partners: Patients should be instructed to refer their sex partners for evaluation, testing, and treatment, if they had sexual contact with the patient during the 60 days preceding onset of symptoms in the patient or diagnosis of chlamydia

Special Considerations:

- *Pregnancy:*
  - Doxycycline and ofloxacin are contraindicated for pregnant women
  - Azithromycin may be safe/effective though the safety and efficacy of azithromycin ◄── use in pregnant and lactating women have not been completely established ◄──
  - Repeat testing, preferably by culture, 3 weeks after completion of therapy with the following regimens is recommended because a) none of these regimens is highly efficacious and b) frequent side effects of erythromycin may discourage patient compliance

- *Recommended Regimens for Pregnant Women*

Erythromycin base..................500 mg orally four times a day for 7 days. OR

Amoxicillin..............................500 mg orally three times a day for 7 days.

- *Alternative Regimens for Pregnant Women*

Erythromycin base..................250 mg orally four times a day for 14 days. OR

Erythromycin ethylsuccinate...800 mg orally four times a day for 7 days, OR

Erythromycin ethylsuccinate...400 mg orally four times a day for 14 days, OR

Azithromycin...........................1 g orally in a single dose.

NOTE: Erythromycin estolate is contraindicated during pregnancy because of drug-related hepatotoxicity. Preliminary data indicate that azithromycin may be safe and effective

GONOCOCCAL INFECTION

DUAL THERAPY FOR GONOCOCCAL AND CHLAMYDIAL INFECTIONS

Patients infected with *N. gonorrhoeae* often are coinfected with *C. trachomatis*; this finding led to the recommendation that patients treated for gonococcal infection also be treated routinely with a regimen effective against uncomplicated genital *C. trachomatis* infection

Uncomplicated Gonococcal Infections of the Cervix, Urethra, and Rectum

- *Recommended Regimens*

Cefixime..................................400 mg orally in a single dose OR

Ceftriaxone.............................125 mg IM in a single dose, OR

Ciprofloxacin..........................500 mg orally in a single dose, OR

Ofloxacin.................................400 mg orally in a single dose, OR

Levofloxocin...........................250 mg orally in a single dose, **AND**

Azithromycin...........................1 g orally in a single dose, OR

Doxycycline.............................100 mg orally twice a day for 7 days

Uncomplicated Gonococcal Infections of the Cervix, Urethra, and Rectum

- **Alternative Regimens**

Spectinomycin........................2 g IM in a single dose. Spectinomycin is effective, but it is expensive and must be injected. It is useful for treatment of patients who cannot tolerate cephalosporins and quinolones

Single-dose cephalosporin.....regimens other than cefritaxone 125 mg IM and cefixime 400 mg include a) ceftizoxime 500 mg IM, b) cefotaxime 500 mg IM, and c) cefoxitin 2 g IM with probenecid 1 g orally

Single-dose quinolone............regimens include gatifloxacin 400 mg orally, lomefloxacin 400 mg orally, and norfloxacin 800 mg orally. None of the regimens appears to offer any advantage over ciprofloxacin or ofloxacin

- Many other antimicrobials are active against *N. gonorrhoeae*
- Azithromycin 2 g orally is effective against uncomplicated gonococcal infection, but it is expensive and causes gastrointestinal distress too often to be recommended for treatment of gonorrhea
- An oral dose of 1 g azithromycin is insufficiently effective and not recommended
- ➤ • Quinolones (Ciprofloxin, Ofloxacin, Levofloxin) should not be used for infections acquired in Asia or the Pacific, including Hawaii

Uncomplicated Gonococcal Infection of the Pharynx

- Gonococcal infections of the pharynx are more difficult to eradicate than infections at urogenital and anorectal sites
- Few antigonococcal regimens can reliably cure such infections >90% of the time
- Although chlamydial coinfection of the pharynx is unusual, coinfection at genital sites sometimes occurs. Therefore, treatment for both gonorrhea and chlamydia is suggested

- **Recommended Regimen**

Ceftriaxone............................125 mg IM in a single dose, OR

Ciprofloxacin.........................500 mg orally in a single dose, PLUS ◄

Azithromycin.........................1 g orally in a single dose, OR

Doxycycline...........................100 mg orally twice a day for 7 days

Management of Sex Partners: All sex partners of patients who have *N. gonorrhea* infection should be evaluated and treated for *N. gonorrhea* and *C. trachomatis* infections if their last sexual contact with the patient was within 60 days before onset of symptoms or diagnosis

Special Considerations:

- Pregnant women should not be treated with quinolones or tetracyclines
- Pregnant women infected with *N. gonorrhoeae* should be treated with a recommended or alternate cephalosporin
- Women who cannot tolerate a cephalosporin should be administered a single 2-g dose of spectinomycin IM
- Either erythromycin or amoxicillin is recommended for treatment of presumptive or diagnosed *C. trachomatis* infection during pregnancy (see CHLAMYDIAL INFECTION, p. 154)

DISEASES CHARACTERIZED BY VAGINAL DISCHARGE

Management of Patients Who Have Vaginal Infections:
- Vaginitis is usually characterized by a vaginal discharge or vulvar itching and irritation; a vaginal odor may be present
- The three diseases most frequently associated with vaginal discharge are trichomoniasis (caused by *T. vaginalis*), BV (caused by a replacement of the normal vaginal flora by an overgrowth of anaerobic microorganisms and *Gardnerella vaginalis*), and candidiasis (usually caused by *Candida albicans*)
- Mucopurulent cervicitis caused by *C. trachomatis* or *N. gonorrhoeae* can sometimes cause vaginal discharge
- Vaginitis is diagnosed by pH and microscopic examination of fresh samples of the discharge
- The pH of the vaginal secretions can be determined by narrow-range pH paper for the elevated pH typical of BV or trichomoniasis (i.e., pH of >4.5)
- One way to examine the discharge is to dilute a sample in one to two drops of 0.9% normal saline solution on one slide and 10% potassium hydroxide (KOH) solution on a second slide. Always prepare saline slide first
- An amine odor detected immediately after applying KOH suggests BV
- A cover slip is placed on each slide, which is then examined under a microscope at low and high-dry power. The motile *T. vaginalis* or the clue cells of BV usually are identified easily in the saline specimen
- The yeast or pseudohyphae of *Candida* species are more easily identified in the KOH specimen
- The presence of objective signs of vulvar inflammation in the absence of vaginal pathogens, along with a minimal amount of discharge, suggests the possibility of mechanical, chemical, allergic, or other noninfectious irritation of the vulva
- Culture for *T. vaginalis* is more sensitive than microscopic examination
- Laboratory testing fails to identify the cause of vaginitis among a minority of women

BACTERIAL VAGINOSIS (BV)

- BV is a clinical syndrome resulting from replacement of the normal H_2O_2 producing *Lactobacillus* sp. in the vagina with high concentrations of anaerobic bacteria (e.g., *Prevotella* sp. and *Mobiluncus* sp.), *G. vaginalis*, and *Mycoplasma hominis*
- BV is the most prevalent cause of vaginal discharge or malodor
- Half of women whose illnesses meet the clinical criteria for BV are asymptomatic
- Treatment of male sex partner has not been beneficial in preventing recurrence

Diagnostic Considerations: BV can be diagnosed by the use of clinical criteria meeting three of the following symptoms or signs:
  a. A homogeneous, white, noninflammatory discharge that smoothly coats the vaginal walls
  b. The presence of clue cells on microscopic examination
  c. A pH of vaginal fluid >4.5
  d. A fishy odor of vaginal discharge before or after addition of 10% KOH (i.e., the whiff test)

Treatment: The principal goal of therapy is to relieve vaginal symptoms and signs of infection. All women with symptoms require treatment, regardless of pregnancy status

> - **BV, Recommended Regimens for Nonpregnant Women**
> Metronidazole...................500 mg orally twice a day for 7 days, OR
> Metronidazole gel............0.75%, one full applicator (5 g) intravaginally, once daily for 5 days OR
> Clindamycin cream............2%, one full applicator (5 g) intravaginally at bedtime for 7 days OR

- Patients should be advised to avoid consuming alcohol during treatment with metronidazole and for 24 hours thereafter. Clindamycin cream is oil-based and might weaken latex condoms and diaphragms

---

- **BV, Alternative Regimens**

Metronidazole.........................2 g orally in a single dose, OR

Clindamycin ovules.................100 mg intravaginally qhs x 3 days

---

Recommended metronidazole regimens are equally efficacious. The vaginal clindamycin cream appears to be less efficacious than the metronidazole regimens

- Metronidazole 2 g single-dose therapy is an alternative regimen because of its lower efficacy for BV
- FDA has approved both metronidazole 750-mg extended release tablets once daily for 7 days and metronidazole gel 0.75% once daily intravaginally for 5 days for treatment of BV. However, data concerning clinical equivalency of these regimens with other regimens have not been published. Some health-care providers remain concerned about the possible teratogenicity of metronidazole, which has been suggested by animal experiments; however, a recent meta-analysis does not indicate teratogenicity in humans

Follow-up:
- Follow-up visits are unnecessary if symptoms resolve. Recurrence is not unusual
- Because treatment of BV in high-risk pregnant women who are asymptomatic might prevent adverse pregnancy outcomes, a follow-up evaluation, at 1 month after completion of treatment, should be considered

Management of Sex Partners: Routine treatment of sex partners is not recommended

Special Considerations:
- *Allergy or Intolerance to the Recommended Therapy:*
  - Clindamycin cream is preferred in case of allergy or intolerance to metronidazole. Metronidazole gel can be considered for patients who do not tolerate systemic metronidazole, but patients allergic to oral metronidazole should not be administered metronidazole vaginally

- *Pregnancy:*
  - BV has been associated with adverse pregnancy outcomes (i.e., premature rupture of the membranes, preterm labor, and preterm birth)
  - Organisms found in increased concentration in BV also are frequently present in postpartum or post-cesarean endometritis
  - Treat all symptomatic pregnant women when diagnosed
  - Treatment of BV in high-risk pregnant women (i.e., those who have previously delivered a premature infant) who are asymptomatic might reduce preterm delivery. However, the optimal treatment regimens have not been established. Some specialists screen and treat those with BV at first prenatal visit
  - The recommended regimen is metronidazole 250 mg orally three times a day for 7 days
  - The alternative regimens are a) metronidazole 2 g orally in a single dose or b) clindamycin 300 mg orally twice a day for 7 days
  - Low-risk pregnant women (i.e., those who previously have not had a premature delivery) who have symptomatic BV should be treated to relieve symptoms. Recommended regimen is metronidazole 250 mg orally three times a day for 7 days
  - Lower doses of medication are recommended for pregnant women to minimize exposure to the fetus. Data are limited concerning the use of metronidazole vaginal gel during pregnancy. Use of clindamycin vaginal cream during pregnancy is not recommended because three randomized trials indicated an increase in the number of preterm deliveries among pregnant women who were treated with this medication

Other: The bacterial flora that characterize BV have been recovered from the endometria and salpinges of women who have PID

TRICHOMONIASIS

Diagnosis:

- Trichomoniasis is caused by the protozoan *T. vaginalis,* easily identified on a wet smear. Most men who are infected do not have symptoms of infection, although a minority of men have nongonococcal urethritis
- Many women do have symptoms of infection, characteristically a diffuse, malodorous, yellow-green discharge with vulvar irritation; many women have fewer symptoms
- Vaginal trichomoniasis might be associated with adverse pregnancy outcomes, particularly premature rupture of the membranes and preterm delivery

Treatment:

- ***Trichomoniasis, Recommended Regimen***
  Metronidazole.........................2 g orally in a single dose

- ***Trichomoniasis, Alternative Regimen***
  Metronidazole.........................500 mg twice a day for 7 days

- Metronidazole is the only oral medication available in the United States
- In randomized clinical trials, the recommended metronidazole regimens have resulted in cure rates of approximately 90% - 95%; ensuring treatment of sex partners might increase the cure rate. Treatment of patients and sex partners results in relief of microbiologic cure, and reduction of transmission
- Discourage use of Metronidazole gel

Follow-up:

- Unnecessary for men and women who become asymptomatic after treatment or who are initially asymptomatic
- Infections with strains of *T. vaginalis* that have diminished susceptibility to metronidazole can occur; however, most of these organisms respond to higher doses of metronidazole
- If treatment failure occurs with either regimen, the patient should be retreated with metronidazole 500 mg twice a day for 7 days
- If treatment failure occurs repeatedly, the patient should be treated with a single, 2g dose of metronidazole once a day for 3-5 days

Management of Sex Partners: Routine Rx recommended avoid intercourse until Rx is complete and both partners are assymptomatic

Special Considerations:

- *Allergy, Intolerance, or Adverse Reactions:* Effective alternatives to therapy with metronidazole are not available. Patients who are allergic to metronidazole can be managed by desensitization
- *Pregnancy:* Patients may be treated with 2 g of metronidazole in a single dose
- *HIV Infection:* Patients who have trichomoniasis and also are infected with HIV should receive the same treatment regimen as those who are HIV negative

VULVOVAGINAL CANDIDIASIS (VVC)

- Vulvovaginal yeast infections are caused by *C. albicans* or, occasionally, by other *Candida* sp., *Torulopsis* sp., or other yeasts
- An estimated 75% of women will have at least one episode of VVC
- A small percentage of women (i.e., probably <5%) experience recurrent VVC
- Typical symptoms of VVC include pruritus and vaginal discharge
- Other symptoms may include vaginal soreness, vulvar burning, dyspareunia, and external dysuria
- None of these symptoms is specific for VVC

Diagnostic Considerations:

- A diagnosis of *Candida* vaginitis is suggested clinically by pruritus and erythema in the vulvo-vaginal area; a white discharge may occur, as may vulvar edema
- The diagnosis can be made in a woman who has signs and symptoms of vaginitis, and when either a) a wet preparation or Gram stain of vaginal discharge demonstrates yeasts or pseudohyphae or b) a culture or other test yields a positive result for a yeast species
- *Candida* vaginitis is associated with a normal vaginal pH (<4.5)
- Use of 10% KOH in wet preparations improves the visualization of yeast and mycelia by disrupting cellular material that might obscure the yeast or pseudohyphae
- Identifying *Candida* by culture in the absence of symptoms should not lead to treatment because 10%-20% of women usually harbor *Candida* sp. and other yeasts in the vagina. VVC can occur concomitantly with STIs or frequently following antibacterial vaginal or systemic therapy

Treatment: Topical formulations effectively treat VVC. The topically applied azole drugs are more effective than nystatin. Treatment with azoles results in relief of symptoms and negative cultures among 80%-90% of patients who complete therapy

- *VVC, Recommended Regimens*
- *Intravaginal agents:*

Butoconazole*............................2% cream 5 g intravaginally for 3 days, **OR**

Butoconazole*............................2% cream 5g (butoconazole 1-sustained release), single vaginal application

Clotrimazole*............................1% cream 5 g intravaginally for 7-14 days, **OR**

Clotrimazole*............................100-mg vaginal tablet for 7 days, **OR**

Clotrimazole*............................100-mg vaginal tablet, two tablets for 3 days, **OR**

Clotrimazole*............................500-mg vaginal tablet, one tablet in a single application, **OR**

Miconazole*............................2% cream 5 g intravaginally for 7 days, **OR**

Miconazole*............................200-mg vaginal suppository, one suppository for 3 days, **OR**

Miconazole*............................100-mg vaginal suppository, one suppository for 7 days, **OR**

Nystatin............................100,000-u vaginal tablet, one tablet for 14 days, **OR**

Tioconazole*............................6.5% ointment 5 g intravaginally in a single application, **OR**

Terconazole*............................0.4% cream 5 g intravaginally for 7 days, **OR**

Terconazole*............................0.8% cream 5 g intravaginally for 3 days, **OR**

Terconazole*............................80-mg vaginal suppository, one suppository for 3 days, **OR**

- *Oral agent:*

Fluconazole............................150-mg oral tablet, one tablet in single dose.

*These creams and suppositories are oil-based and may weaken latex condoms and diaphragms

- *VVC, Alternative Regimens*
- The ease of administering oral agents is an advantage over topical therapies
- However, the potential for toxicity associated with using a systemic drug, particularly ketoconazole, must be considered

Follow-up: Patients should be instructed to return for follow-up visits only if symptoms persist or recur

Management of Sex Partners: None; VVC usually is not acquired through sexual intercourse

Special Considerations:

- *Pregnancy:* VVC often occurs during pregnancy. Only topical azole therapies should be used to treat pregnant women. Of those treatments that have been investigated for use during pregnancy, the most effective are butoconazole, clotrimazole, miconazole, and terconazole. Many experts recommend 7 days of therapy during pregnancy
- *HIV Infection:* Studies are in progress to confirm an alleged increase in incidence of VVC in HIV-infected women

PELVIC INFLAMMATORY DISEASE (PID) (see Table 13.1, page 35)

- PID comprises a spectrum of inflammatory disorders of the upper female genital tract, including any combination of endometritis, salpingitis, tuboovarian abscess, and pelvic peritonitis
- Sexually transmitted organisms, especially *N. gonorrhoeae* and *C. trachomatis*, are implicated in most cases; however, microorganisms that can be part of the vaginal flora (e.g., anaerobes, *G. vaginalis, H. influenzae*, enteric gram negative rods, and *Streptococcus agalactiae*) also can cause PID
- In addition, CMV, *M. hominis* and *U. urealyticum* may also be etiologic agents

Diagnostic Considerations: See complete *2002 CDC Guidelines (www.cdc.gov)*. Empiric treatment should be initiated in sexually active young women and others at risk for STIs if all the following **minimum criteria** are present and no other cause(s) for the illness can be identified:

- Uterine/adnexal tenderness or
- Cervical motion tenderness

Treatment: Must provide empiric, broad-spectrum coverage of likely pathogens
Antimicrobial coverage should include *N. gonorrhea, C. trachomatis*, anaerobes, gram-negative facultative bacteria, and streptococci

- *Criteria for HOSPITALIZATION based on observational data and theoretical concerns:*
  - Surgical emergencies such as appendicitis cannot be excluded
  - Patient is pregnant
  - Patient does not respond clinically to oral antimicrobial therapy
  - Patient is unable to follow or tolerate an outpatient oral regimen
  - Patient has severe illness, nausea and vomiting, or high fever
  - Patient has a tuboovarian abscess; or

Most clinicians favor at least 24 hours of direct inpatient observation for patients who have tuboovarian abscesses. After that, parenteral therapy should have reduced the risk of abcess progression or rupture

- *PID, Parenteral Regimen A*

Cefotetan....................................2 g IV every 12 hours, **OR**
Cefoxitin.....................................2 g IV every 6 hours, **PLUS**
Doxycycline..............................100 mg IV or orally every 12 hours

- Because of pain associated with infusion, doxycycline should be administered orally when possible, even when the patient is hospitalized
- Both oral and IV administration of doxycycline provide similar bioavailability
- When tuboovarian abscess is present, many health-care providers use clindamycin or metronidazole with doxycycline for continued therapy rather than doxycycline alone, because it provides more effective anaerobic coverage

- **PID, Parenteral Regimen B**

Clindamycin..........................900 mg IV every 8 hours, **PLUS**

Gentamicin..........................loading dose IV or IM (2 mg/kg of body weight) followed by a maintenance dose (1.5 mg/kg) every 8 hours. Single daily dosing may be substituted.

- Although use of a single daily dose of gentamicin has not been evaluated for the treatment of PID, it is efficacious in analogous situations
- Parenteral therapy may be discontinued 24 hours after a patient improves clinically, and continuing oral therapy should consist of doxycycline 100 mg orally twice a day or clindamycin 450 mg orally four times a day to complete a total of 14 days of therapy
- When tuboovarian abscess is present, many healthcare providers use clindamycin for continued therapy rather than doxycycline because clindamycin provides more effective anaerobic coverage

---

- **PID, Alternative Parenteral Regimens:** Limited data support the use of other parenteral regimens, but the following three regimens have been investigated in at least one clinical trial, and they have broad-spectrum coverage.

Ofloxacin..........................400 mg IV every 12 hours, OR Levofloxacin 500 mg IV once daily with or without metronidazole 500 mg IV every 8 hours **OR**

Ampicillin/Sulbactam............3 g IV every 6 hours, PLUS doxycycline 100 mg IV / orally every 12 hours **OR**

Oral Treatment: The following regimens provide coverage against the frequent etiologic agents of PID, but evidence from clinical trials supporting their use is limited. Patients who do not respond to oral therapy within 72 hours should be reevaluated to confirm the diagnosis and be administered parenteral therapy on either an outpatient or inpatient basis.

- **PID, Oral Regimen A**

Ofloxacin..........................400 mg orally twice a day for 14 days, **PLUS**

Levofloxacin..........................500 mg daily for 14 days, WITH or WITHOUT ◄━━

Metronidazole..........................500 mg orally twice a day for 14 days.

- **PID, Oral Regimen B**

Ceftriaxone..........................250 mg IM once, **OR**

Cefoxitin..........................2 g IM plus probenecid, 1 g orally in a single dose concurrently once, **OR**

Other parenteral third-generation cephalosporin (e.g.,ceftizoxime or cefotaxime), **PLUS**

Doxycycline..........................100 mg orally twice a day for 14 days with or without metronidazole 500 mg orally twice daily for 14 days.

Follow-up:
- Patients receiving oral or parenteral therapy should demonstrate substantial clinical improvement (i.e., defervescence; reduction in direct or rebound abdominal tenderness; and reduction in uterine, adnexal, and cervical motion tenderness) within 3 days after initiation of therapy
- Patients who do not improve within 3 days usually require additional diagnostic tests, surgical intervention, or both
- If the health-care provider prescribes outpatient oral or parenteral therapy, a follow-up examination should be performed within 72 hours

Special Considerations:
- *Pregnancy:* Pregnant women who have suspected PID should be hospitalized and treated with parenteral antibiotics.

HUMAN PAPILLOMAVIRUS INFECTION (HPV)

Genital Warts

- More than 30 types of HPV can infect the genital tract. Most HPV infections are asymptomatic, subclinical, or unrecognized. Visible genital warts usually are caused by HPV types 6 or 11. Other HPV types in the anogenital region (i.e., types 16, 18, 31, 33, and 35) have been strongly associated with cervical dysplasia
- No data support the use of type-specific HPV nucleic acid tests in the routine diagnosis or management of visible genital warts
- HPV types 6 and 11 also can cause warts on the uterine cervix and in the vagina, urethra, and anus; these warts are sometimes symptomatic
- HPV types 6 and 11 are associated rarely with invasive squamous cell carcinoma of the external genitalia
- HPV types 16, 18, 31, 33, and 35 are found occasionally in visible genital warts and have been associated with external genital (i.e., vulvar, penile, and anal) squamous intraepithelial neoplasia (i.e., squamous cell carcinoma in situ, bowenoid papulosis, erythroplasia of Queyrat, or Bowen's disease of the genitalia). These HPV types have been associated with vaginal, anal, and cervical intraepithelial dysplasia and squamous cell carcinoma. Patients who have visible genital warts can be infected simultaneously with multiple HPV types

Treatment:

- The primary goal of treating visible genital warts is the removal of symptomatic warts
- Treatment can induce wart-free periods in most patients. Genital warts often are asymptomatic
- **No evidence indicates that currently available treatments eradicate or affect the natural history of HPV infection.** The removal of warts may or may not decrease infectivity
- If left untreated, visible genital warts may resolve on their own, remain unchanged, or increase in size or number. No evidence indicates that treatment of visible warts affects the development of cervical cancer

Regimens:

- Treatment of genital warts should be guided by the patient's preference, the available resources, and the experience of the health-care provider.
- None of the available treatments is superior to other treatments, and no single treatment is ideal for all circumstances. The treatment modality should be changed if a patient has not improved substantially after three provider-administered treatments or if warts have not completely cleared after six treatments
- Providers should be knowledgeable about, and have available, at least one patient-applied and one provider-administered treatment

- ***External Genital Warts, Recommended Treatments:***
- *Patient-Applied*

Podofilox............................0.5% solution or gel.

- Patients may apply podofilox solution with a cotton swab, or podofilox gel with a finger, to visible genital warts twice a day for 3 days, followed by 4 days of no therapy
- This cycle may be repeated as necessary for a total of four cycles
- The total wart area treated should not exceed 10 cm^2, and a total volume of podofilox should not exceed 0.5 mL per day
- If possible, the health-care provider should apply the initial treatment to demonstrate the proper application technique and identify which warts should be treated. The safety

of podofilox during pregnancy has not been established. **OR**

Imiquimod.............................5% cream.

- Patients should apply imiquimod cream with a finger at bedtime, three times a week for as long as 16 weeks
- The treatment area should be washed with mild soap and water 6-10 hours after the application
- Many patients may be clear of warts by 8-10 weeks or sooner
- The safety of imiquimod during pregnancy has not been established

- *Provider-Administered:*
  Cryotherapy with liquid nitrogen or cryoprobe. Repeat applications every 1 to 2 weeks **OR** Trichloroacetic acid (TCA) or BCA 80%-90%. May place petroleum jelly around wart to reduce spread of medication to normal mucosa. Apply a small amount only to warts and allow to dry, at which time a white "frosting" develops; powder with talc or NaHCO$_3$ to remove unreacted acid if an excess amount is applied. Repeat weekly if necessary. **OR**
  Podophyllin resin...................10%-25% in tincture of benzoin.
- A small amount should be applied to each wart and allowed to air dry
- To avoid the possibility of complications associated with systemic absorption and toxicity, some experts recommend that application be limited to <0.5 mL of podophyllin or <10 cm^2 of warts per session
- Some experts suggest that the preparation should be thoroughly washed off 1-4 hours after application to reduce local irritation. Repeat weekly if necessary
- *The safety of podophyllin during pregnancy has not been established*
- *Surgical removal* by tangential scissor excision, tangential shave excision, curettage, or electrosurgery

- **External Genital Warts, Alternative Treatments (Provider administered)**
Intra-lesional interferon **OR**
Laser surgery

- *Cervical Warts*
For women who have exophytic cervical warts, high-grade squamous intraepithelial lesions (SIL) must be excluded before treatment is begun. Management of exophytic cervical warts should include consultation with an expert

- *Vaginal Warts, Recommended Treatment*
Cryotherapy with liquid nitrogen. The use of a cryoprobe in the vagina is not recommended because of the risk for vaginal perforation and fistula formation. **OR**
TCA or BCA 80%-90% applied only to warts. Repeat weekly if necessary.

- *Urethral Meatus Warts, Recommended Treatment*
Cryotherapy with liquid nitrogen **OR**
Podophyllin 10%-25% in tincture of benzoin. The treatment area must be dry before contact with normal mucosa. Podophyllin must be applied weekly if necessary. *The safety of podophyllin during pregnancy has not been established.*

- *Anal Warts, Recommended Treatment*

Cryotherapy with liquid nitrogen **OR**

TCA or BCA 80%-90% applied to warts. Apply a small amount only to warts and allow to dry, at which time a white "frosting" develops; powder with talc or sodium bicarbonate (i.e., baking soda) to remove unreacted acid if an excess amount is applied. Repeat weekly if necessary. May place petroleum jelly around wart to reduce spread of medication to normal mucosa **OR**

Surgical removal

- Management of warts on rectal mucosa should be referred to an expert

Follow-up: After visible genital warts have cleared, a follow-up is not mandatory

Management of Sex Partners: None. Examination of sex partners is not necessary for the management of genital warts because the role of reinfection is probably minimal and, in the absence of curative therapy, treatment to reduce transmission is not realistic

Special Considerations:

- *Pregnancy:* Imiquimod, podophyllin, and podofilox should not be used during pregnancy. Because genital warts can proliferate and become friable during pregnancy, many experts advocate their removal during pregnancy. HPV types 6 and 11 can cause laryngeal papillomatosis in infants and children. Vaginal delivery not contraindicated unless lesion size obstructive in labor (rare). The route of transmission (i.e., transplacental, perinatal, or postnatal) is not completely understood

VACCINE-PREVENTABLE STIs

One of the most effective means of preventing the transmission of STIs is preexposure immunization. Currently licensed vaccines for the prevention of STIs include those for hepatitis A and hepatitis B. Clinical development and trials are underway for vaccines against a number of other STIs, including HIV and HSV. As more vaccines become available, immunization possibly will become one of the most widespread methods used to prevent STIs

ECTOPARASITIC INFECTIONS

PEDICULOSIS PUBIS

Patients who have pediculosis pubis (i.e., pubic lice) usually seek medical attention because of pruritus. Such patients also usually notice lice or nits on their pubic hair

Treatment:

- *Pediculosis Pubis, Recommended Regimens*

Permethrin..........................1% creme rinse applied to affected areas and washed off after 10 minutes **OR**

Lindane................................1% shampoo applied for 4 minutes to the affected area, and then thoroughly washed off. This regimen is not recommended for pregnant or lactating women or for children aged <2 yrs **OR**

Pyrethrins with piperonyl butoxide applied to the affected area and washed off after 10 minutes.

Other Management Considerations:

- The recommended regimens should not be applied to the eyes. Pediculosis of the eyelashes should be treated by applying occlusive ophthalmic ointment to the eyelid margins twice a day for 10 days
- Bedding and clothing should be decontaminated (either machine-washed and machine-dried using the heat cycle or drycleaned) or removed from body contact for at least 72 hrs
- Fumigation of living areas is not necessary

Follow-up: Patients should be evaluated after 1 week if symptoms persist. Retreatment may be necessary if lice are found or if eggs are observed at the hairskin junction. Patients who do not respond to one of the recommended regimens should be retreated with an alternative regimen

Management of Sex Partners: Sex partners within the last month should be treated

Special Considerations:
- ***Pregnancy:*** Pregnant and lactating women should be treated with either permethrin or pyrethrins with piperonyl butoxide

SCABIES

- Predominant symptoms is pruritus; sensitization takes several weeks to develop; pruritus might occur within 24 hours after a subsequent reinfestation
- Scabies in adults may be sexually transmitted, although scabies in children usually is not

- ***Scabies, Recommended Regimen***
  Permethrin cream.................(5%) applied to all areas of the body from the neck down and washed off after 8-14 hours.

- ***Scabies, Alternative Regimens***
  Lindane....................................(1%) 1 oz. of lotion or 30 g of cream applied thinly to all areas of the body from the neck down and thoroughly washed off after 8 hours **OR**
  Ivermectin...............................200 mg/kg orally, repeated in 2 weeks
  - Lindane should not be used immediately after a bath, and it should not be used by a) persons who have extensive dermatitis, b) pregnant or lactating women, and c) children aged <2 years.

Other Management Considerations: Bedding and clothing should be decontaminated (i.e., either machine-washed or machine-dried using the hot cycle or dry-cleaned) or removed from body contact for at least 72 hours. Fumigation of living areas is unnecessary

Follow-up: Pruritus may persist for several weeks. Some experts recommend retreatment after 1 week for patients who are still symptomatic; other experts recommend retreatment only if live mites are observed. Patients who do not respond should be retreated with an alternative regimen

Management of Sex Partners and Household Contacts: Both sexual and close personal or household contacts within the preceding month should be examined and treated

SEXUAL ASSAULT AND STIs: Adults and Adolescents

Evaluation for Sexually Transmitted Infections
- ***Initial Examination*** - (See inside back cover)
- ***Follow-up Examination after Assault***
  - Examination for STIs should be repeated 2 weeks after assault (see inside back cover)
  - Serologic tests for syphilis and HIV infection should be repeated 6, 12, and 24 weeks after the assault if initial test results were negative
- ***Prophylaxis:*** Many experts recommend routine preventive therapy after a sexual assault. The prophylactic regimen suggested is on inside back cover
- An empiric antimicrobial regimen for chlamydia, gonorrhea, trichomonas, and BV should be administered (See inside back cover)

Other Management Considerations:

At the initial examination and, if indicated, at follow-up, patients should be counseled about:

- Risk for pregnancy and possible use of emergency contraception
- Symptoms of STIs and the need for immediate examination if symptoms occur
- Abstinence from sexual intercourse until STI prophylactic treatment is completed

Risk for Acquiring HIV Infection:

- Although HIV antibody seroconversion has been reported among persons whose only known risk factor was sexual assault or sexual abuse, the risk for acquiring HIV infection through sexual assault is low and depends on many factors
- These factors may include the type of sexual intercourse (i.e., oral, vaginal, or anal); presence of oral, vaginal or anal trauma; site of exposure to ejaculate; viral load in ejaculate; and presence of an STI

HIV INFECTION

OraQuick, a rapid test (40-60 minutes) was approved by the FDA in November, 2002. ◄
For entire guidelines see www.aidsinfo.nih.gov ◄

Proper management of HIV infection involves a complex array of behavioral, pyschosocial, and medical services. This information should not be a substitute for referral to a health-care provider or facility experienced in caring for HIV-infected patients. The following hotlines may provide excellent information and referrals for provider and patient:

```
CDC AIDS Treatment Information Service.........1-800-HIV-0440 (1-800-448-0440)
    e-mail to: atis@hivatis.org & www.hivatis.org
CDC AIDS Clinical Trials Information Service...1-800-TRIALS-A (1-800-874-2572)
    e-mailto: actis@actis.org
    International.............1-301-519-0459
For general information and referrals to local facilities:
CDC National AIDS Hotline.................................1-800-342-AIDS (1-800-342-2437)
    Spanish......................1-800-344-7432
CDC National AIDS Clearinghouse......................1-800-458-5231
CDC Division of HIV/AIDS Prevention.................www.cdc.gov/hiv
Post exposure prophylaxis PEP...........................1-888-HIV-4911
```

Pregnancy: All pregnant women should be offered HIV testing as early in pregnancy as possible. This recommendation is particularly important because of the available treatments for reducing the likelihood of perinatal transmission and maintaining the health of the woman. HIV-infected women should be informed specifically about the risk for perinatal infection. Current evidence indicates that 15%-25% of infants born to untreated HIV-infected mothers are infected with HIV; the virus also can be transmitted from an infected mother by breastfeeding. Zidovudine (ZDV) reduces the risk for HIV transmission to the infant from approximately 25% to 8% if administered to women during the later stage of pregnancy and during labor and to infants for the first 6 weeks of life. Therefore, **ZDV TREATMENT SHOULD BE OFFERED TO ALL HIV-INFECTED PREGNANT WOMEN.** Most women in the U.S. now receive triple therapy during pregnancy not just ZDV. In the United States, HIV-infected women should be advised not to breast-feed their infants. In other countries, the reduced risk of death from malnutrition, diarrheal disease, or other infections may outweigh the risk of contracting HIV.

Insufficient information is available regarding the safety of ZDV or other antiretroviral drugs during early pregnancy; however, on the basis of the ACTG-076 protocol, ZDV is indicated for the prevention of maternal-fetal HIV transmission as part of a regimen that includes oral ZDV at 14-34 weeks of gestation, intravenous (IV) ZDV during labor, and ZDV syrup to the neonate after birth.

WHO MEDICAL ELIGIBILITY CRITERIA FOR STARTING CONTRACEPTIVE METHODS (2000)

The table on the following pages summarizes the latest World Health Organization (WHO) medical eligibility criteria for starting contraceptives. These criteria are also the basis for the checklists throughout *Managing Contraception*. These criteria are for the most part evidence-based. References are available through the World Health Organization

WHO categories for temporary methods:

WHO 1   **Can use** the method. No restriction on use.

WHO 2   **Can use** the method. Advantages generally outweigh theoretical or proven risks. If method is chosen, more than usual follow-up may be needed.

WHO 3   **Should not use** the method unless clinician makes clinical judgment that the patient can safely use it. **Theoretical or proven risks usually outweigh the advantages** of method. Method of last choice, for which regular monitoring may be needed.

WHO 4   **Should not use** the method. Condition represents an unacceptable health risk if method is used.

Simplified 2-category system for temporary methods

To make clinical judgment, the WHO 4-category classification system can be simplified into a 2-category system.

WHO Category	With Clinical Judgment	With Limited Clinical Judgment
1	Use the method in any circumstances	Use the method
2	Generally use the method	
3	Use of the method not usually recommended unless other, more appropriate methods are not available or acceptable	Do not use the method
4	Method not to be used	

NOTE: In the pages that follow, Category 3 and 4 conditions are shaded to indicate the method should not be provided where clinical judgment is limited.

WHO MEDICAL ELIGIBILITY CRITERIA FOR STARTING CONTRACEPTIVE METHODS (2001)

CONDITION	Combined OCs	Combined Injectables	Progestin-Only OCs	Depo-Provera NET EN	Norplant Implants	Condoms	Spermicides	Diaphragm	TCU-380A IUD	LNG IUD
PERSONAL CHARACTERISTICS & REPRODUCTIVE HISTORY										
Pregnant	NA	NA	NA	NA	NA	NA	NA	NA	NA	NA
Age	Menarche to <40=1	Menarche to <40=1	Menarche to <18=1	Menarche to <18=2	Menarche to <40=1	Menarche to <40=1	Menarche to <40=1	Menarche to <40=1	<20=2	<20=2
	≥40=2	≥40=2	18-45=1	18-45=1	18-45=1				≥20=1	≥20=1
			>45=1	>45=2	>45=1					
Parity a) nulliparous	1	1	1	1	1	1	1	1	2	2
b) parous	1	1	1	1	1	1	1	1	1	1
Breastfeeding < 6 weeks PP	4	4	3	3	3					
≥6 weeks to 6 months PP primarily breastfeeding	3	3	1	1	1					
≥ 6 months PP	2	2	1	1	1					
Postpartum < 21 days	3	3	1	1	1			NA		
≥ 21 days	1	1	1	1	1				<48 hrs 3 / 48h-<4wks 3 / ≥4 wks 1	<48 hrs 3 / 48h-<4wks 3 / >4 wks 1
Puerperal Sepsis									4	4
Post-abortion 1st trimester	1	1	1	1	1	1	1	1	1	1
2nd trimester	1	1	1	1	1	1	1	1	2	2
Immediate post septic AB	1	1	1	1	1	1	1	1	4	4
Past ectopic pregnancy	1	1	2	1	1	1	1	1	1	1

For women older than 45 there are concerns regarding hypo-estrogenic effect of DMPA on bone mass.

There is concern that the neonate may be at risk of exposure to steroid hormones during the first 6 weeks. POCs may be one of the few types of methods available and accessible to breastfeeding women immediately postpartum.

History of pelvic surgery	1		1	1	1	1	1	1	1	1
Smoking: Less than age 35	2	2		1	1	1	1	1	1	2
Age ≥ 35 < 15 cigarettes/day	3	2		3	1	1	1	1	1	2
Age ≥ 35 ≥ 15 cigarettes/day	4	3		4	1	1	1	1	1	2
Obesity ≥ 30 kg/m² BMI	2	2		2	1	1	1	1	1	2
CARDIOVASCULAR DISEASE										
Multiple risk factors for CAD (older age, smoking, diabetes, HBP)	3 or 4	3 or 4	2	3	2	1	1	1	1	1	2
HBP Hx HBP, BP can't be evaluated	3	3	2	2	2	1	1	1	1	1	2
HBP adequately controlled	3	3	1	2	1	1	1	1	1	1	1
BP systolic 140-159 or Diastolic 90-99	3	3	1	2	1	1	1	1	1	1	1
BP systolic > 160 or Diastolic 100	4	4	2	3	2	1	1	1	1	1	2
Vascular disease	4	4	2	3	2	1	1	1	1	1	2
HBP during pregnancy, BP now normal	2	2	1	1	1	1	1	1	1	1	1
Deep vein thrombosis/pulmonary embolism											
a) History of DVT/PE	4	4	2	2	2	1	1	1	1	1	2
b) Current DVT/PE	4	4	3	3	3	1	1	1	1	1	3
c) Family History (first-degree relatives)	2	2	1	1	1	1	1	1	1	1	1
d) Major surgery with prolonged immobilization	4	4	2	2	2	1	1	1	1	1	2
e) Major surgery without prolonged immobilizaton	2	2	1	1	1	1	1	1	1	1	1
f) Minor surgery without immobilization	1	1	1	1	1	1	1	1	1	1	1

When multiple major risk factors exist, risk of CV disease may increase substantially. Some POCs may increase risk of thrombosis although this risk is substantially less than with COCs.

A3

WHO MEDICAL ELIGIBILITY CRITERIA FOR STARTING CONTRACEPTIVE METHODS (CONTINUED)

CONDITION	Combined OCs	Combined Injectables	Progestin-Only OCs	Depo-Provera NET EN	Norplant Implants	Condoms	Spermicides	Diaphragm	TCu-380A IUD	LNG IUD	
Superficial venous thrombosis											
a) varicose veins	1	1	1	1	1	1	1	1	1	1	← Varicose Veins are not risk factors for DVT/PE
b) superficial thrombophlebitis	2	2	1	1	1	1	1	1	1	1	
Current & history of ischemic heart disease	4	4	2/3*	3	2/3	1	1	1	1	2/3	← There is concern regarding reduced HDL levels among POC users. Some POCs may increase the risk of arterial thrombosis, although this increase is substantially less than with COCs.
Stroke (history of CVA)	4	4	2/3	3	2/3	1	1	1	1	2	
Known hyperlipidemia	2* or 3*	2 or 3	2	2	2	1	1	1	1	2	
Valvular heart disease uncomplicated	2	2	1	1	1	1	1	1	1	1	
Valvular heart disease complicated	4	4	1	2	1	1	1	1	2	2	
NEUROLOGIC CONDITIONS											
Headaches											
a) non-migraine (mild or severe)	1/2	1/2	1/1	1/1	1/1	1	1	1	1	1/1	
b) migraine < 35; no focal neurologic symptoms	2/3	2/3	1/2	2/2	2/2	1	1	1	1	2/2	← New evidence: Among women with migraines, women who also have focal neurologic symptoms have a higher risk of stroke than those without focal neurologic symptoms. In addition, among women with migraines, those who use COCs have a 2 to 4-fold increased risk of stroke compared with women who do not use COCs.
c) migraine ≥ 35; no focal neurologic symptoms	3/4	3/4	1/2	2/2	2/2	1	1	1	1	2/2	
d) migraine with focal neurologic Sx (any age)	4/4	4/4	2/3	2/3	2/3	1	1	1	1	2/3	
Epilepsy	1	1	1	1	3	1	1	1	1	1	
REPRODUCTIVE TRACT INFECTIONS & DISORDERS											
Irregular without heavy bleeding	1	1	2	2	2	1	1	1	1	1/1	
Heavy or prolonged vaginal bleeding (regular or irregular)	1	1	2	2	2	1	1	1	2	1/2	
Unexplained vaginal bleeding. Suspicious for serious underlying condition. Before evaluation.	2	2	2	3	3	1	1	1	4/2	4/2	

* Initiation: 2 and Continuation: 3 expressed as 2/3 (I/C)
** If distinction is made between levels of severity of a condition it is expressed as 2 or 3

Condition												
Endometriosis	1	1	1	1	1	1	1	1	2	1		← Copper IUD may worsen dysmenorrhea associated with endometriosis
Benign ovarian tumors (including cysts)	1	1	1	1	1	1	1	1	1	1		
Severe dysmenorrhea	1	1	1	1	1	1	1	2	1			
Benign gestational trophoblastic disease	1	1	1	1	1	1	1	3	3			
Malignant gestational trophoblastic disease	1	1	1	1	1	1	4	4	4			
Cervical ectropion	1	1	1	1	1	1	1	1	1			
Cervical intraepithelial neoplasia (CIN)	2	2	1	2	2	1	1	1	2			← There is some concern that COCs enhance the progression of CIN to invasive disease, particularly with long-term use
Cervical cancer (awaiting treatment)	2	2	2	2	2	1	1	4*/2	4/2			
Undiagnosed breast mass	2	2	2	2	2	1	1	1	2			
Benign breast disease	1	1	1	1	1	1	1	1	1			
Family history of breast cancer	1	1	1	1	1	1	1	1	1			
Breast cancer (current)	4	4	4	4	4	1	1	1	4			← Breast cancer is hormonally sensitive, and the prognosis of women with current or recent breast cancer may worsen with COC or POC use
Past breast cancer; No current disease for 5 years	3	3	3	3	3	1	1	1	3			
Endometrial cancer	1	1	1	1	1	1	1	4/2	4/2			
Ovarian cancer	1	1	1	1	1	1	1	3/2	3/2			
Uterine fibroids without distortion of uterine cavity	1	1	1	1	1	1	1	2	2			
Uterine fibroids with distortion of uterine cavity	1	1	1	1	1	1	1	4	4			

A5

WHO MEDICAL ELIGIBILITY CRITERIA FOR STARTING CONTRACEPTIVE METHODS (CONTINUED)

CONDITION	Combined OCs	Combined Injectables	Progestin-Only OCs	Depo-Provera NET EN	Norplant Implants	Condoms	Spermicides	Diaphragm	TCu-380A IUD	LNG IUD	
Past history PID (no current STI risk factors) with subsequent pregnancy	1	1	1	1	1	1	1	1	1/1	1/1	
Past history PID (no current STI risk factors) without subsequent pregnancy	1	1	1	1	1	1	1	1	2/2	2/2	In women at low risk of STIs, IUD insertion poses little risk of PID. Current risk of STIs and desire for future pregnancy are relevant considerations
Current PID (or within last 3 months)	1	1	1	1	1	1	1	1	4¹/3	4¹/3	
STI: current or past 3 months (including purulent cervicitis)	1	1	1	1	1	1	1	1	4	4	
Vaginitis without purulent cervicitis	1	1	1	1	1	1	1	1	2	2	
Increased risk of STIs	1	1	1	1	1	1	1	1	3	3	
HIV/AIDS											
High risk of HIV	1	1	1	1	1	1	2	1	3**	3**	Women at high risk of HIV are also at high risk of other STIs
HIV-positive	1	1	1	1	1	1	2	1	3**	3**	
AIDS	1	1	1	1	1	1	2	1	3**	3**	
ENDOCRINE CONDITIONS											
History gestational diabetes	1	1	1	1	1	1	1	1	1	1	
Non-insulin dependent diabetes (non-vascular disease)	2	2	2	2	2	1	1	1	1	1	
Insulin dependent diabetes (non-vascular disease)	2	2	2	2	2	1	1	1	1	1	
Diabetic nephropathy/retinopathy/neuropathy	3/4	3/4	2	3	2	1	1	1	1	2	There is concern about the possible negative effect of DMPA on lipid metabolism, possibly affecting the progression of nephropathy, retinopathy or other vascular disease
Other vascular disease; diabetes of > 20 years	3/4	3/4	2	3	2	1	1	1	1	2	

* Initiation: 4 and Continuation: 3 expressed as 4/3 (I/C).

** Many experts, including the author of the IUD chapter in the next edition of Contraceptive Technology, Dr. David Grimes, argue that there are no data demonstrating risks of IUDs in these categories

CONDITION	Combined OCs	Combined Injectables	Progestin-Only OCs	Depo-Provera NET EN	Norplant Implants	Condoms	Spermicides	Diaphragm	TCu-380A IUD	LNG IUD
Thyroid: simple goiter	1	1	1	1	1	1	1	1	1	1
Hyperthyroid	1	1	1	1	1	1	1	1	1	1
Hypothyroid	1	1	1	1	1	1	1	1	1	1
GASTROINTESTINAL CONDITIONS										
Symptomatic gall bladder disease post cholecystectomy	2	2	2	2	2	1	1	1	1	2
Symptomatic gall bladder disease medically treated	3	2	2	2	2	1	1	1	1	2
Symptomatic gall bladder disease - current	3	2	2	2	2	1	1	1	1	2
Asymptomatic gall bladder disease	2	2	2	2	2	1	1	1	1	2
History of pregnancy-related cholestasis	2	2	1	1	1	1	1	1	1	1
Past COC-related cholestasis	3	2	2	2	2	1	1	1	1	2
Viral hepatitis active	4	3/4*	3	3	3	1	1	1	1	3
Viral hepatitis carrier	1	1	1	1	1	1	1	1	1	1
Cirrhosis mild compensated	3	2	2	2	2	1	1	1	1	2
Benign hepatic adenoma	4	3	3	3	3	1	1	1	1	3
Malignant liver tumor (hepatoma)	4	3/4	3	3	3	1	1	1	1	3

*Initiation: 3 and Continuation: 4 expressed as 3/4 (I/C)

COCs may cause small increased risk of gall bladder disease. There is also concern that COCs may worsen existing gallbladder disease

COCs are metabolized by liver and use may adversely affect women whose liver function is already compromised. There is concern about the hormonal load associated with POC use, but it is less than for COCs

WHO MEDICAL ELIGIBILITY CRITERIA FOR STARTING CONTRACEPTIVE METHODS (CONTINUED)

CONDITION	Combined OCs	Combined Injectables	Progestin-Only OCs	Depo-Provera NET EN	Norplant Implants	Condoms	Spermicides	Diaphragm	TCu-380A IUD	LNG IUD
ANEMIAS										
Thalassemia	1	1	1	1	1	1	1	1	2	1
Sickle cell disease	2	2	1	1	1	1	1	1	2	1
Iron deficiency anemia	1	1	1	1	1	1	1	1	2	1
DRUG INTERACTIONS										
Rifampicine & griseofulvin	3	3	3	2	3	1	1	1	1	1
Anticonvulsants: Phenytoin, barbiturates carbamazepine, primidone	3	3	3	2	3	1	1	1	1	1
Other antibiotics (other than rifampicin/griseofulvin)	NA	1	1	1	1	1	1	1	1	1
Allergy to latex	NA	NA	NA	NA	NA	3	1	3	NA	NA

Although the interaction between commonly used liver enzyme inducers and COCs is not harmful to women, it is likely to reduce the efficacy of COCs. Use of other contraceptives should be encouraged for women who are long-term users of any of these drugs. Whether increasing the hormone dose of COCs is of benefit remains unclear.

HISTORY OF CONTRACEPTION AND POPULATION GROWTH

"We have not inherited the earth from our grandparents, we have borrowed it from our grandchildren."
—PROFESSOR JOHN GUILLEBAUD-ATTRIBUTED TO THE ANCIENT CHINESE

2001	Ortho Evra Patch and NuvaRing approved	
2000	RU486 (mifepristone), Lunelle and Mirena approved by FDA	
1999	World population hits **6 billion** (this billion took 12 years)	1999 - 6 billion (10/12/99!!)
1997	FDA approves Emergency Contraceptive Pills	
1994	Plastic (polyurethane) condom for men (Avanti)	
1993	FDA approves polyurethane (plastic) female condom (Reality)	
1993	Creinin and Darney describe medical abortion using methotrexate	
1992	FDA approves Depo-Provera (DMPA) injections	
1990	FDA approves Norplant implants	
1988	Copper T 380-A IUD marketing begins, 5 years after FDA approval	
1987	World population reaches **5 billion** (this billion took 12 years)	1987 - 5 billion
1983	FDA approves Copper T 380-A and the Today sponge	
1982	Baulieu describes medical abortion using mifepristone	
1981	First documented case of HIV/AIDS	
1981	Garret Hardin writes "nobody ever dies of overpopulation" after 500,000 die from flooding of an overcrowded East Bengal River delta	
1975	World population reaches **4 billion** (this billion took 15 years)	1975 - 4 billion
1974	Al Yuzpe describes emergency contraception using Ovral pills	
1973	FDA approved progestin-only pills (minipills)	
1973	U.S. Supreme Court abortion decision (Roe v Wade & Doe v Bolton)	
1965	U.S. Supreme Court Griswold v. CT, overturns anti-birth control laws in most states	
1965	U.S. Agency of International Development initiates Population Program	
1960	Food and Drug Administration approves combined oral contraceptives	
1960	World population reaches **3 billion** (this billion took 30 years)	
1942	American Birth Control League renamed Planned Parenthood	
1937	AMA ends longstanding opposition to contraception	
1936	German gynecologist Friedrich Wilde describes first cervical cap (fitted from a wax impression)	
1930-31	Knaus (Austria) and Ogino (Japan) develop rhythm method	
1930	World population now **2 billion** (this billion took 100 years)	1960 - 3 billion
1930	Pope Pius XI virulently attacks both contraception & abortion	
1927	Novak (Hopkins) describes suction as means of performing an abortion	
1916	Margaret Sanger opens first Amercian birth control clinic in Brooklyn, NY	
1914	Margaret Sanger coins word "birth control"	
1912	Sadie Sachs post-abortion death affects Margaret Sanger profoundly	
1909	German surgeon Richard Richter reports success with silkworm-gut shaped into a ring	
1893	First vasectomy by Harrison in London	
1882	First contraceptive clinic established in Amsterdam	1930 - 2 billion
1880	First tubal ligation	
1873	Comstock Act: classifies birth control devices and information as obscene	
1839	Charles Goodyear discovers vulcanization technology; quickly leads to rubber condoms	
1830	World population reaches **1 billion** (this billion took 6 million years)	
1798	Thomas Robert Malthus proposes dismal economic theory that population growth eventually will exceed the ability of the earth to provide food, resulting in starvation	1800 - 1 billion
Late 1770s	Casanova popularizes condoms for infection control and contraception	
1 AD	World population reaches **250 million**, abstinence (particularly postpartum), withdrawal, lactation, stones in camels, lemons for mechanical and spermicidal effect, abortion using molokeeia (same stem used today), homosexuality and polygamy	
	1 AD - 250 million	

Special thanks to Andrea Tone at Georgia Tech

American College of Obstetrics and Gynecologists (ACOG). Emergency oral contraception. ACOG Practice Patterns 1996 (Dec. no. 3).

Arevalo M, Jennings V, Sinai I. Efficacy of a new method of family planning: the Standard Days Method. Contraception. 2001; 65:333-338.

Artz, L, Demand M, Pulley LV, Posner SF, Macaluso M. Predictors of difficulty inserting the female condom. Contraception 65, 2002:151-157.

Association for Voluntary Surgical Contraception. Postpartum IUD insertion: Clinical and programatic guidelines (monograph) 1994 (AVSC has changed name to Engender Health).

Audet MC, Moreau M, Koltun WD, Waldbaum AS, Shangold G, Fisher AC, Creasy MD. Evaluation of contraceptive efficacy and cycle control of a transdermal contraceptive patch vs. an oral contraceptive: a randomized controlled trial. JAMA. 285;2001:2347-2354.

Ballagh SA. Sterilization in the office: the concept is now a reality. Contraceptive Technology Reports. February, 2003 supplement to the newsletter, Contraceptive Technology Update.

Berel V, Hermon C, Kay C, Hannaford P, Darby S, Reeves G. Mortality associated with oral contraceptive use: 25 year follow-up of cohort of 46,000 women from Royal College of General Practitioners' oral contraceptive study; Br Med J 1999: 918:96-100.

Berlex Laboratories, Inc. YASMIN prescribing information: Physician Labeling and Patient Instructions; June, 2001.

Brache V, Alvarez-Sanchez F, Faundes A, Tejada AS, Cochon L. Ovarian endocrine function through five years of continuous treatment with Norplant subdermal contraceptive implants. Contraception 1990;41:169.

Briggs GG, Freeman RK, Yaffe SJ. Drugs in Pregnancy and Lactation, Fifth edition. Lippincott Williams & Wilkins, Philadelphia. 1998.

Canto-DeCetina TEC, Canto P, Luna MO. Effect of counseling to improve compliance in Mexican women receiving depot-medroxyprogesterone acetate. Contraception 63; 2001: 143-146.

Centers for Disease Control and Prevention. 1998 Guidelines for treatment of sexually transmitted diseases. MMWR 1998:47(No. RR-1): 1-118.

Centers for Disease Control Cancer and Steroid Hormone Study. Long-term oral contraceptive use and the risk of breast cancer. JAMA. 1983; 249:1591-1595.

Colditz GA, Rosner BA, et al. Risk factors for breast cancer according to family history of breast cancer. J Natl Cancer Inst. 1996;88:365-371.

Collaborative Group on Hormonal Factors in Breast Cancer. Breast cancer and hormonal contraceptives: collaborative reanalysis of individual data on 53,297 women with breast cancer and 100,239 women without breast cancer from epidemiological studies. Lancet 1996; 347:1713-1727.
A10

Coutinho EM with Segal SJ. Is Menstruation Obsolete? Oxford University Press; Oxford; New York; 1999.

Creinin MD, Burke AE. Methotrexate and misoprostol for early abortion: a multicenter trial. Acceptablity. Contraception 1996;54:19-22.

Creinin MD, Vittinghoff E, Schaff E, Klaisle C, Darney PD, Dean C. Medical abortion with oral methotrexate and vaginal misoprostol. Obstet Gynecol 1997;90:611-5.

Cromer BA, Blair JM, Mahan JD, Zibners L, Naumovski Z. A prospective comparison of bone density in adolescent girls receiving depo-medroxyprogesteroneacetate (Depo-Provera), levonorgestrel (Norplant), or oral contraceptives. J Pediatr 1996;129:671-6.

Croxatto HB, Diaz S, Pavez M, et al. Plasma progesterone levels during long-term treatment with levonorgestrel silastic implants. Acta Endocrinol 1982;101:307-11.

Curtis et al. Contraception for Women in Selected Circumstances. Obstetrics and Gynecology, June 2002; 99 (6):1100-1112

de Abood M, de Castillo 2, Guerrero E, Espino M, Austin KL. Effect of Depo-Provera or Microgynon in the painful crises of sickle-cell anemia patients. Contraception 56; 1997:313.

Cundy T, Evans M, Roberts H, Wattie D, Ames R, Reid IR. Bone density in women receiving depot medroxyprogesterone acetate for contraception. BMJ 1991; 303: 13-16.

Diaz J, Bahamondes L, Monteiro I, Peta C, Hildalgo MM, Arce XE. Acceptability and performance of the levonorgestrel-releasing intrauterine system (Mirena) in Campinas, Brazil. Contraception 2000; 62: 59-61.

Farley TM, Rosénberg MS, Rowe PJ, Chen SH, Meirck O. Intrauterine devices and pelvic inflammatory disease: an international perspective. Lancet 1992; 339: 785-88.

Feldblum PJ, Morrison CS, Roddy RE, Cates W Jr. The effectiveness of barrier methods of contraception in preventing the spread of HIV. AIDS 1995;9 (suppl A):585-93.

Finer LB, Henshaw SK. Abortion incidence and service in the United States in 2000. Perspectives on Sexual and Reproductive Health 2003; 35(1): 6-15.

Ford K, Labbok M. Contraceptive use during lactation in the United States: an update. American Institute of Public Health 1987; 77: 79-81.

Fraser SI, Affandi B, Croxatto HB, et al. Norplant consensus statement and background paper. Turku, Finland: Leiras Oy International, 1997.

Frezieres RG, Walsh TL, Nelson AL, Clark VA, Coulson AH: Breakage and acceptability of a polyurethane condom: A randomized controlled study. Fam Plann Perspect 1998;30;73-8.

Goldstein M, Girardi S. Vasectomy and vasectomy reversal. Curr Thera Endocrinol Metab 1997;6:317-80.

Grabrick DH, Hartmann LC, Cerhan FR, Vierkant RA, Therneau TM, et al. Risk of Breast Cancer with Oral Contraceptive Use in Women With a Family History of Breast Cancer. JAMA; 284:1791-1798.

Gray RH, Campbell OM, Zacur H, Labbok MH, MacRae SL. Postpartum return of ovarian activity in non-breastfeeding women monitored by urinary assays. J Clin Endocrinol Metab 1987;64:645-50.

Grimes DA. Health benefits of oral contraception: update on endometrial cancer prevention. The Contraception Report 2001;12(3):4-7.

Grimes DA. Modern IUDs: an update. The Contraception Report; November, 1998.

Grimes DA. Should first-time OC users be screened for genetic thrombophilia? The Contraception Report; 10:1, p.p. 9-11; March 1999.

Grimes DA. Transdermal contraceptive patch awaiting US approval. The Contraception Report; 12(4):12-14.

Guillebaud J. Contraception, your questions answered, 3rd edition. London, Churchill Livingstone, 1999.

Guillebaud J. Personal communication; October 14, 2001.

Hafner DW, Schwartz P. What I've Learned about Sex. A Perigee Book: New York: The Berkeley Publishing Group, 1998.

Hakim-Elahi E, Tovell HMM, Burnhill MS. Complications of first-trimester abortion: a report of 170,000 cases. Obstet Gynecol 1990;76:129.

Hall PE. New once-a-month injectable contraceptives, with particular reference to Cyclofem/Cyclo-Provera. Int. J Gynaecol Obstet 1998; 62: S43-S56.

Henshaw SK. Unintended pregnancy in the United States. Fam Plann Perspect 1998;30:24-9, 46.

Hatcher RA, Trussell J, Stewart F, Cates W Jr, Stewart GK, Guest F, Kowal D. *Contraceptive Technology*, 17th ed. New York NY, Ardent Media, 1998

Hogue CJR, Cates W Jr, Tietze C. The effects of induced abortion on subsequent reproduction. The Johns Hopkins University School of Hygiene and Public Health. Epidemiol Rev 1982;4:66

International Planned Parenthood Federation Handbook 1997.

Jones RK, Dorroch JE, Henshaw SK. Patterns with socioeconomic characterics of women obtaining abortions in 2000-2001. Perspectives in Sexual and Reproductive Health 2002,34: 226-235.

Kaunitz AM. personal communications; December 28, 1998 and February 24, 1999.

Kaunitz AM, Garceau RJ, Cromie MA. Comparative safety, efficacy, and cycle control of Lunelle monthly contraceptive injection (medroxyprogesterone acetate and estradiol cypionate injectable suspension) and Ortho-Novum 7/7/7 oral contraceptive (norethindrone/ethinyl estradiol triphasic). Contraception 1999; 60(4):179-187.

Kennedy KI, Trussell J. Postpartum contraception and lactation. IN Hatcher RA, Trussell J, Stewart F et al: Contraceptive Technology, 17th ed.; New York: Ardent Media Inc; 1998: 592-4. [The same data are presented in the Family Health International Module for the teaching of Lactational Amenorrhea]

Kjos SL, Peters RK, Xiang A, Duncan T, Schaefer U, Buchanan TA. Contraception and the risk of type 2 diabetes mellitus in Latina women with prior gestational diabetes mellitus. JAMA 1998; 280: 533-38.

Klavon SL, Grubb G. Insertion site complications during the first year of Norplant use. Contraception 1990;41:27.

Krattenmacher R. Drospirenone: pharmacology and pharmacokinetics of a unique progestogen. Contraception 2000; 62:29-38.

Lawson ML, Macaluso M, Duerr A, Hortin G, Hammond KR, Blackwell R, Artz L and ◄ Bloom A. Partner characteristics, intensity of intercourse, and semen exposure during use of the female condom. Am J Epidemiol; 2003; 157:282-288.

Lipnick RJ, Buring JE, Hennekens CH, et al. Oral contraceptives and breast cancer: a prospective cohort study. JAMA. 1986; 255:58-61.

Marguiles R, Miller L. Increased depot medroxyprogesterone acetate use increases family planning program pharmaceutical supply costs. Contraception 2001 (63):147-149.

Miller L, Grice J. Intradermal proximal field block: an innovative anesthetic technique for levonorgestrel implant removal. Obstet Gynecol 1998;91:294-297.

Monteiro I, Bahamondes L, Diaz J, Perotti M, Petta C. Therapeutic use of levonorgestrel- ◄ releasing intrauterine systems in women with menorrhagia: a pilot study. Contraception 65; 2002; 325-328.

Mulders TMT, Dieben TOM. Use of the novel combined contraceptive vaginal ring NuvaRing for ovulation inhibition. *Fertility and Sterility* 2001; 75:865-870.

Murray PP, Stadel BV, Schlesselman JJ. Oral contraceptive use in women with a family history of breast cancer. Obstet Gynecol. 1989; 73:977-983.

Narod ST. The Hereditary Ovarian Cancer Clinical Study Group. Oral contraceptives and the risk of hereditary ovarian cancer. N Engl J Med 1998;339;424-8.

Narod ST. et al. Lancet 357 [9267]: 1467-70, 2001.

Ness RB, Grisso JA, Klapper J, et al. Risk of ovarian cancer in relation to estrogen and progestin dose and use characteristics of oral contraceptives. Am J Epidemiol 2000;152: 233-241.

O'Hanley K, Huber DH. Postpartum IUDs: keys for success. Contraception 1992; 45: 351-361.

Peipert JF, Gutman J. Oral contraceptive risk assessment: a survey of 247 educated women. Obstet Gynecol 1993;82:112-7.

Peterson HB, Jeng G, Folger SG et al for the U.S. Collaborative Review of Sterilization Working Group. N Engl J Med 2000; 343:1681-7.

Peterson HB, Pollack AE, Warshaw JS. Tubal sterilization. In: Rock JA, Thompson JD, eds. TeLinde's Operative Gynecology. 8th ed. Philadelphia: Lippincott-Raven, 1997:541-5.

Phelps RH, Schaff EA, Fielding SL. Mifepristone abortion in minors. Contraception 2001; 64: 339-343.

Polaneczky M, Guarnaccia, Alon J, Wiley J. Early experience with the contraceptive use of depot medroxyprogesterone acetate in an inner-city clinic population. Family Planning Perspectives 1996; 28: 174-178.

Raudaskoski TH, Lahti EI, Kauppila AJ, Apaja-Sarkkinen MA, Laatikainen TJ. Transdermal estrogen with a levonorgestrel-releasing intrauterine device for climacteric complaints: clinical and endometrial responses. Am J Obstet Gynecol 1995;172:114-9.

Redmond G, Godwin AJ, Olson W, Lippman JS. Use of placebo controls in an oral contraceptive trial: methodological issues and adverse event incidence. Contraception 1999;60:81-5.

Roumen FJ, Apter D, Mulders TM, et al. Efficacy, tolerability and acceptability of a novel contraceptive vaginal ring releasing etonogestrel and ethinyl estradiol. Hum Reprod 2001;16:469-475.

Schwallie PC, Assenzo JR. Contraceptive use-efficacy study initializing medroxyprogesterone acetate administered as an intramuscular injection once every 90 days. Fertil Steril 1973; 24(5):331-339. ◄——

Segal SJ. Is menstruation obsolete? Lecture in Atlanta, Georgia. November 1, 2001.

Shelton JD. Repeat emergency contraception: facing our fears. Contraception 66;2002:15-17.

Silvestre L, Dubois C, Renault M, Rezvani Y, Baulieu E, Ulmann A. Voluntary interruption of pregnancy with mifepristone (RU-486) and a prostaglandin analogue. N Engl J Med 1990; 322:645-8.

Shulman LP, Oleen-Burkey M, Willke RJ. Patient acceptability and satisfaction with Lunelle monthly contraceptive injection (medroxyprogesterone acetate and estradiol cypionate injectable suspension). Contraception 1999;60(4):215-222.

Smith TW. Personal communication to James Trussell. December 13, 1993.

Speroff L, Darney PD. A Clinical Guide for Contraception. Third Edition. Lippincott Williams & Wilkins; Philadelphia; 2001.

Speroff L, Glass RH, Kase NG. Clinical Gynecologic Endocrinology and Infertility. Sixth Edition. 1999; Lipincott Williams & Wilkins; Baltimore, Maryland.

Speroff L. The perimenospaausal transition: maximizing preventive health care. In: Mooney B, Daughtery J, eds. Midlife Women's Health Sourcebook. Atlanta: American Health Consultants, 1995.

Stewart FH, Harper CC, Ellertson CE, Grimes DA, Sawyer GF, Trussell J. Clinical breast and pelvic examination requirements for hormonal contraception: Current practice vs. evidence. JAMA 2001;285:2232-2239.

Task Force on Postovulatory Methods of Fertility Regulation. Randomized controlled trial of levonorgestrel versus the Yuzpe regimen of combined oral contraceptives for emergency contraception. Lancet 1998;352:420-33.

The Alan Guttmacher Institute. Sex and America's Teenagers. New York and Washington: 1994.

The Hereditary Ovarian Cancer Clinical Study Group. Oral contraceptives and the risk of hereditary ovarian cancer. N Engl J Med 1998;339;424-8.

Trussell J, Leveque JA, Koenig JD, et al. The economic value of contraception: a comparison of 15 methods. Am J Public Health 1995;85:494-503.

Trussell J, Stewart F, Guest F, Hatcher RA. Emergency contraceptive pills: a simple proposal to reduce unintended pregnancies. Fam Plann Perspect 1992;24:269-73.

Valle RF, Carignan CS, Wright TC, et al. Tissue response to STOP microcoil transcervical permanent contraceptive device: results from a prehysterectomy study. Fertil Steril 2001; 76: 974

Von Hertzen H, Piaggio G, Ding J et al. Low dose Mifepristone and two regimens of levonorgestrel for emergency contraception: a WHO multicentre randomised trial. Lancet 2002; 360: 1803-10.

Walsh T, Grimes D, Frezieres R, Nelson A, Bernstein L, Coulson A, Bernstein G. Randomized controlled trial of prophylactic antibiotics before insertion of intrauterine devices. *Lancet* 1998:351;1005-1008.

Westoff C, Kerns J, Morroni C, Cushman LF, Tiezzi L, Murphy PA. Quick Start: a novel contraceptive initiation method. Contraception 66; 2002:141-145.

White MK, Ory HW, Rooks JB, Rochat RW. Intrauterine device termination rates and menstrual cycle day of insertion. Obstet Gynecol 1980; 55:220-4.

Willett WC, Green A, Stampfer MJ, Speizer FE, Colditz GA, Rosner B, Monson RR, Stason W, Hennekens CH. Relative and absolute risks of coronary heart disease among women who smoke cigarettes. New Eng J Med 317:1303, 1987.

World Health Organization, Department of Reproductive Health and Research. Improving Access to Quality Care in Family Planning: Medical Eligibility Criteria for Contraceptive Use. Second Edition. Geneva. 2000.

World Health Organization. WHO Taskforce Postovulatory Methods of Fertility Regulation. Lancet Aug 8, 1998.

Writing Group for the Women's Health Initiative. Risks and benefits of estrogen plus progestin in healthy postmenopausal women. JAMA 2002; 288: 321-333.

Zieman M, Guillebaud J, Weisberg E, Shangold G, Fisher A, Creasy G. Integrated summary of contraceptive efficacy with the Ortho Evra transdermal system. Fertility and Sterility Supplement; September, 2001. S19

TOPIC	WEBSITE
Abortion	www.naral.org
	www.prochoice.org
Adolescent Reproductive Health	www.teenpregnancy.org
	www.ama-assn.org/adolhlth/adolhlth.htm
	www.advocatesforyouth.org
Contraception	www.conrad.org
	www.who.int (World Health Organization Precautions)
	www.contraceptiononline.org/contrareport
	www.managingcontraception.com
	www.ippf.org
	www.plannedparenthood.org
	www.reproline.jhu.edu
	www.avsc.org/avsc
Counseling	www.gmhc.org
Education	www.siecus.org
	www.cdc.gov
Emergency Contraception	www.not-2-late.com (ec.princeton.edu)
HIV/AIDS/STIs	www.CritPath.Org/aric
	www.cdc.gov/hiv
	www.cdc.gov/nchstp/dstd/dstdp.htm
Managing Contraception	www.managingcontraception.com
Menopause	www.menopause.org
	www.osteo.org
Natural Family Planning	www.canfp.org
(Fertility Awareness)	www.familyplanning.net
	www.ccli.org
Population Organizations	www.popcouncil.org
	www.prb.org
	www.undp.org/popin/infoserv.htm
	www.population.org/homepage.htm
Professional Organizations	www.acog.org
	www.arhp.org
	www.fda.gov
	www.fhi.org
	www.jsi.com
	www.NPWH.org
	www.obgyn.net
	www.pathfind.org
	www.plannedparenthood.org
	www.who.int
Reproductive Health Research	www.agi-usa.org
	www.kff.org
	www.fhi.org

SPANISH/ESPAÑOL	ENGLISH/INGLES
• Abstinencia	• Abstinence
• Amamantar a Su Bebe	• Breast-feeding
• Tapa Cervical	• Cervical Cap
• Retraer el pene antes de ejecular	• Coitus Interruptus (Withdrawal)
• Injecciones Combinadas	• Combined Injectables
• La Pildora	• Combined Oral Contraceptives (COCs)
• Condones parce hombres	• Condoms for Men
• Condones para Mujeres	• Condoms for Women
• La "T" o Dispositivo do Cobre	• Copper T 380-A
• Injecciones de Depo-Provera	• Depo-Provera
• El Diafragma	• Diaphragm
• Contraceptivo de Emergencia	• Emergency Contraception
• Consciente Sobre Metodos de Fertilidad	• Fertility Awareness Methods
• Espuma Contraceptiva	• Foam
• Metodos para el Futuro	• Future Methods
• Dispositivos	• IUDs
• Gelatina Anticonceptiva	• Jellies
• El Dispositivo de "Levo Norgestrel"	• Levonorgestrel IUD
• Implantes de NORPLANT	• Norplant Implant
• El Dispositivo de "Progestasert"	• Progestasert IUD
• Contraceptives de Progesterona Solamente	• Progestin-Only Contraceptives
• Pildoras de Progesterona Solamente	• Progestin-Only Pills (POPs)
• RU-486 (Mifepristone)	• RU-486 (Mifepristone)
• Espermicidas	• Spermicides
• Ligadura o Estirilizacion de las Trompas	• Tubal Sterilization
• Tela Anticonceptiva	• Vaginal contraceptive film
• Vasectomia	• Vasectomy
• Todos los dispositivos	• All other IUDs at this time

<u>NOTE:</u> Final pages of
Appendix (A18 - A26)
are at very end of book

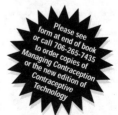

Please see
form at end of book
or call 706-265-7435
to order copies of
Managing Contraception
or the new edition of
Contraceptive
Technology

SPANISH EDITION

INCLUDES:

- Anita Nelson, MD is the senior author for this 2000-2001 edition
- Updated information on the vaginal ring
- LUNELLE–the once-a-month shot
- Plan B, the new progestin-only emergency contraceptive pill
- STI's (CDC guidelines)
- Depo-Provera (what procedure to follow if late getting injection)
- 8 pages in color of all oral contraceptives
- Menstrual cycle physiology
- and MUCH MORE!
- Dedicated to the first woman president of ACOG, Dr. Luella Klein

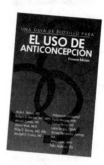

Written for all sexually active women and men

A warm and friendly book for people who really want to inform themselves about the contraceptives they are using or considering.

- Advantages and disadvantages of each contraceptive
- 8 full color photo pages of all oral contraceptive pills
- What to do if emergency ("morning after") contra-ception is needed
- Lubricants that can and cannot be used with condoms
- Extensive information on sexually transmitted infections
- Flow charts explaining *what to do if one or two pills are missed*, if spotting occurs on pills, if late for a Depo-Provera injection or if switching from pills to menopausal estrogen replacement therapy

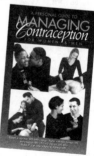

12 full-page photos of 4 couples making the book
- More attractive to scan
- Less dense
- More user-friendly

For college students & all young adults (18-22)

Welcome to the exciting world of Sexual Etiquette!

This book contains stories, resources, ideas, and other valuable tools to help you successfully navigate the often confusing world of relationships and sexuality.

Through this book, we aim to provide you with information to help you prevent the possibly negative and harmful side of sexuality so that you can enjoy the pleasurable and beautiful side of sexuality and make decisions that are right for you.

Here's a glimpse of what you will find in the NEW Sexual Etiquette 101 & More, 4th Edition:

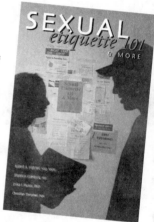

- ▶ Long-distance relationships
- ▶ Outercourse (what it is and why you may love it)
- ▶ Selecting a method of contraception that will work for you
- ▶ Why condoms are so important
- ▶ What to do if you are sexually assaulted
- ▶ Making sexual behavior mutual & consensual
- ▶ What it takes for abstinence to work
- ▶ Contemporary HIV/AIDS issues
- ▶ Breaking-up
- ▶ Communication tips throughout
- ▶ All of these important issues AND MORE!

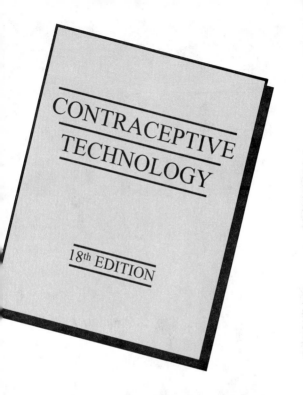

familia
planificación

una guía para
la salud reproductiva
y la anticoncepción

{la planificación familiar}

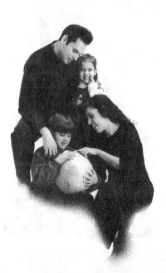

Robert A. Hatcher, MD, MPH

Erika I. Pluhar, PhD

Miriam Zieman, MD

Anita Nelson, MD

Philip Darney, MD, MSc

Peter W. Hatcher, MD

Traducción al espanol:

Carlos Moisa, MD

Myriam Hernández-Jennings, MA

Claudia Burnham, BS

Jay Miranda, BA

A guide to Managing Contraception for Women and Men–
For the General Public...All in Spanish.

		Quantity	Total
...cket Guide to Managing Contraception 2003-2004 (for clinicians)			
1-99	10.00 ea	_____	_____
100-199	9.00 ea	_____	_____
200-299	8.00 ea	_____	_____
300	6.00 ea	_____	_____
...lanificación Familiar (for general Spanish speaking public)			
1-99	16.95 ea	_____	_____
100-199	12.95 ea	_____	_____
...sonal Guide to Managing Contraception for Women and Men (for the general public)			
1-99	14.95 ea	_____	_____
100-199	11.95 ea	_____	_____
...nething Nice Calendar			
1-9	15.00 ea	_____	_____
10-499	12.00 ea	_____	_____
...traceptive Technology - 17th Edition			
1-24	39.95 ea	_____	_____
25-50	35.00 ea	_____	_____
51-100	30.00 ea	_____	_____
...ual Etiquette 101 & More			
1-24	5.95 ea	_____	_____
25-499	2.50 ea	_____	_____
500-999	2.00 ea	_____	_____
...st for Excellence			
1-24	4.95 ea	_____	_____
25-499	2.00 ea	_____	_____
500-999	1.50 ea	_____	_____
...ergency Contraceptive Kits			
10 (minimum)	35.00	_____	_____
11-100	3.00 ea	_____	_____
101-500	2.50 ea	_____	_____
...nd Trust: A Child's Legacy			
	13.95 ea	_____	_____
...vices & Desires - A History of Contraceptives in America			
	30.00 ea	_____	_____
...thel: Mustang Ranch and Its Women			
	14.95 ea	_____	_____
...Menstruation Obsolete?			
	24.00 ea	_____	_____
	Sub total		_____
	Georgia locations add 7% sales tax		_____
	15% Shipping		_____
	Add $1 Handling Fee		_____
	Total Enclosed		_____

...accept check or credit cards: VISA, MasterCard, Discover & American Express

...edit Card No. _____ Expiration Date: _____

...nature: _____ (Required)

...IP TO: Name: _____

...ganization: _____

...dress: _____ Zip _____

...one No. _____ Fax No. _____

...mail _____

...il or Fax this ORDER FORM with your payment to:
...dging the Gap Communications • P.O. Box 888 • Dawsonville, GA 30534
...ke checks payable to Bridging the Gap Communications
...one: (706) 265-7435 • Fax: (706) 265-6009 • www.ManagingContraception.com
...ail: btg@ProjectPlanetCorp.com
...ANK YOU! (CALL FOR SPECIAL PRICES ON LARGER QUANTITIES & INTERNATIONAL SHIPPING)   JS 04/03

BRIDGING THE GAP COMMUNICATIONS, INC.

COLOR PHOTOS
of Combined and Progestin-Only Oral Contraceptives
www.managingcontraception.com ←

The eight color pages of pills are organized as follows:

Color photos of pills from lowest to highest estrogen dose..........A18-A24

- Progestin-only pills with **no estrogen**: Micronor, NOR-QD, and Ovrette

- Lowest estrogen pills with **20 micrograms** of the estrogen, ethinyl estradiol: Alesse, Levlite, LoEstrin 1/20, and Mircette

- All of the **30- and 35-microgram** pills (all ethinyl estradiol)

- All of the **phasic** pills

- Highest estrogen pills, with **50 micrograms** of estrogen (ethinyl estradiol OR mestranol). Mestranol is converted in the body to ethinyl estradiol; 50 mcg of mestranol is equivalent to 35 mcg of ethinyl estradiol

* There are prominent horizontal or vertical parallel lines ("equal signs") between pills which are pharmacologically exactly the same. The color and packaging of pills dispensed in clinics may differ from pills in pharmacies.

Pill Warning Signals...A25
The "ACHES" method of teaching women on pills what to watch out for and the problems a clinician or counselor should think about if one of these symptoms develops.

Pills you can prescribe as emergency contraceptive pills...............A26

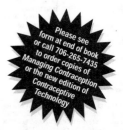

Please see form at end of book or call 706-265-7435 to order copies of Managing Contraception or the new edition of Contraceptive Technology

PROGESTIN - ONLY PILLS

**MICRONOR® TABLETS
28-DAY REGIMEN**
(0.35 mg norethindrone) (lime green)
Ortho-McNeil

=

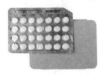

NOR-QD® TABLETS
(0.35 mg norethindrone) (yellow)
Watson

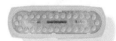

OVRETTE® TABLETS
(0.075 mg norgestrel) (yellow)
Wyeth-Ayerst

COMBINED PILLS - 20 microgram PILLS

=

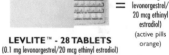

LEVLITE™ - 28 TABLETS
(0.1 mg levonorgestrel/20 mcg ethinyl estradiol)
(active pills pink)
Berlex

=

AVIANE
(0.1 mg
levonorgestrel/
20 mcg ethinyl
estradiol)
(active pills
orange)

ALESSE - 28 TABLETS
(0.1 mg levonorgestrel/20 mcg ethinyl estradiol)
(active pills pink)
Wyeth-Ayerst

LOESTRIN® FE 1/20
(1 mg norethindrone acetate/20 mcg ethinyl
estradiol/75 mg ferrous fumarate [7d])
(active pills white)
Parke-Davis

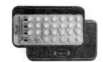

MIRCETTE - 28 TABLETS
(0.15 mg desogestrel/ 20 mcg ethinyl estradiol X 21 (white)/
placebo X 2 (green)/10 mcg ethinyl estradiol X 5 (yellow)
Organon

COMBINED PILLS - 30 microgram PILLS

 =

LEVLEN® 28 TABLETS
(0.15 mg levonorgestrel/30 mcg ethinyl estradiol)
(active pills light orange)
Berlex

LO/OVRAL®-28 TABLETS
(0.3 mg norgestrel/30 mcg ethinyl estradiol)
(active pills white)
Wyeth-Ayerst

‖

‖

NORDETTE®-28 TABLETS
(0.15 mg levonorgestrel/30 mcg ethinyl estradiol)
(active pills light orange)
Monarch

LOW-OGESTREL - 28
(0.3 mg norgestrel/30 mcg ethinyl estradiol)
(active pills white)
Watson

‖

‖

SEASONALE
(0.15 mg levonorgestrel/30 mcg ethinyl estradiol)
84 active pills followed by 7 placebo pills

=

LEVORA TABLETS
(0.15 mg levonorgestrel/30 mcg ethinyl estradiol)
(active pills white)
Watson

DESOGEN® 28 TABLETS
(0.15 mg desogestrel/30 mcg ethinyl estradiol)
(active pills white)
Organon

LOESTRIN® 21 1.5/30
(1.5 mg norethindrone acetate/ 30 mcg ethinyl estradiol)
(active pills green)
Parke-Davis

‖

**ORTHO-CEPT® TABLETS
28-DAY REGIMEN**
(0.15 mg desogestrel/30 mcg ethinyl estradiol)
(active pills orange)
Ortho-McNeil

YASMIN 28 TABLETS
(3.0 mg drospirenone/30 mcg ethinyl estradiol)
(active pills yellow)
Berlex

A20

COMBINED PILLS - 35 microgram PILLS

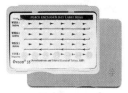

OVCON® 35 28-DAY
(0.4 mg norethindrone/35 mcg ethinyl estradiol)
(active pills peach)
Warner-Chilcott

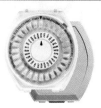

**ORTHO-CYCLEN®
28 TABLETS**
(0.25 mg norgestimate/35 mcg ethinyl estradiol)
(active pills blue)
Ortho-McNeil

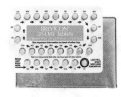

**BREVICON®
28-DAY TABLETS**
(0.5 mg norethindrone/35 mcg ethinyl estradiol)
(active pills blue)
Watson

=

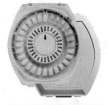

**MODICON® TABLETS
28-DAY REGIMEN**
(0.5 mg norethindrone/35 mcg ethinyl estradiol)
(active pills white)
Ortho-McNeil

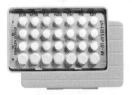

DEMULEN® 1/35-28
(1 mg ethynodiol diacetate/35 mcg ethinyl estradiol)
(active pills white)
Pharmacia

=

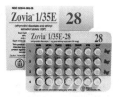

ZOVIA® 1/35E–28
(1 mg ethynodiol diacetate/35 mcg ethinyl estradiol)
(active pills light pink)
Watson

A21

COMBINED PILLS - 35 microgram PILLS (continued)

 =

NORETHIN 1/35E–28
(1 mg norethindrone/35 mcg ethinyl estradiol)
(active pills white)
Shire

**ORTHO-NOVUM® 1/35
28 TABLETS**
(1 mg norethindrone/35 mcg ethinyl estradiol)
(active pills peach)
Ortho-McNeil

ǁ

ǁ

 =

NORINYL® 1+35 28-DAY TABLETS
(1 mg norethindrone/35 mcg ethinyl estradiol)
(active pills yellow-green)
Watson

NECON 1/35-28
(1 mg norethindrone/35 mcg ethinyl estradiol)
(active pills dark yellow)
Watson

COMBINED PILLS - PHASIC PILLS

**ORTHO TRI-CYCLEN®
LO - 28 TABLETS**
(norgestimate/ethinyl estradiol)
0.18 mg/25 mcg (7d) (white),
0.215 mg/25 mcg (7d) (light blue),
0.25 mg/25 mcg (7d) (dark blue)
remaining 7 placebo pills are green
Ortho-McNeil

CYCLESSA
(desogestrel/ethinyl estradiol–triphasic regimen)
0.1 mg/25 mcg (7d) (light yellow)
0.125 mg/25 mcg (7d) (orange)
0.150 mg/25 mcg (7d) (red)
Organon

 = =

TRIVORA®
(levonorgestrel/ethinyl
estradiol–triphasic regimen)
0.050 mg/30 mcg (6d), 0.075
mg/40 mcg (5d),
0.125 mg/30 mcg (10d) (pink)
Watson

**TRIPHASIL®-
28 TABLETS**
(levonorgestrel/ethinyl
estradiol–triphasic regimen)
0.050 mg/30 mcg (6d) (brown),
0.075 mg/40 mcg (5d) (white),
0.125 mg/30 mcg (10d)
(light yellow)
Wyeth-Ayerst

**TRI-LEVLEN®
28 TABLETS**
(levonorgestrel/ethinyl estradiol–
triphasic regimen)
0.050 mg/30 mcg (6d) (brown),
0.075 mg/40 mcg (5d) (white),
0.125 mg/30 mcg (10d)
(light yellow)
Berlex

**ORTHO-NOVUM® 10/11
28 TABLETS**
(norethindrone/ethinyl estradiol)
0.5 mg/35 mcg (10d) (white),
1 mg/35 mcg (11d) (peach)
Ortho-McNeil

JENEST 28 TABLETS
(norethindrone/ethinyl estradiol)
0.5 mg/35 mcg (7d) (white),
1 mg/35 mcg (14d) (peach)
Organon

**TRI-NORINYL®
28-DAY TABLETS**
(norethindrone/ethinyl estradiol)
0.5 mg/35 mcg (7d) (blue),
1 mg/35 mcg (9d) (yellow-green),
0.5 mg/35 mcg (5d) (blue)
Watson

**ORTHO-NOVUM® 7/7/7
28 TABLETS**
(norethindrone/ethinyl estradiol)
0.5 mg/35 mcg (7d) (white),
0.75 mg/35 mcg (7d) (light peach),
1 mg/35 mcg (7d) (peach)
Ortho-McNeil

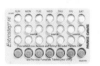

**ORTHO TRI-CYCLEN®
28 TABLETS**
(norgestimate/ethinyl estradiol)
0.18 mg/35 mcg (7d) (white),
0.215 mg/35 mcg (7d) (light blue),
0.25 mg/35 mcg (7d) (blue)
Ortho-McNeil

**ESTROSTEP® FE
28 TABLETS**
(norethindrone acetate/ethinyl estradiol)
1 mg/20 mcg (5d) (white triangular),
1 mg/30 mcg (7d) (white square),
1 mg/35 mcg (9d), 75 mg ferrous
fumarate (7d) (white round)
Parke-Davis

A23

COMBINED PILLS - 50 microgram PILLS

Pills with 50 micrograms of mestranol are not as strong as pills with 50 micrograms of ethinyl estradiol

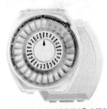

**ORTHO-NOVUM® 1/50
28 TABLETS**
(1 mg norethindrone/50 mcg mestranol)
(active pills yellow)
Ortho-McNeil

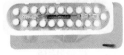

OVRAL - 21 TABLETS
(0.5 mg norgestrel/50 mcg ethinyl estradiol)
(active pills white)
Wyeth-Ayerst

= **OGESTREL**
Watson

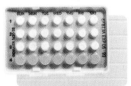

DEMULEN® 1/50-28
(1 mg ethynodiol diacetate/50 mcg ethinyl estradiol)
(active pills white)

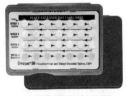

OVCON® 50 28-DAY
(1 mg norethindrone/50 mcg ethinyl estradiol)
(active pills yellow)
Warner-Chilcott

PILL WARNING SIGNALS

Pills have been studied extensively and are very safe. However, very rarely pills lead to serious problems. Here are the warning signals to watch out for while using pills. These warning signals spell out the word **ACHES**. If you have one of these symptoms, it may or may not be related to pill use. You need to check with your clinician as soon as possible. The problems that could possibly be related to using pills are as follows:

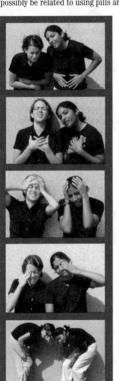

ABDOMINAL PAIN
- Blood clot in the pelvis or liver
- Benign liver tumor or gall bladder disease

CHEST PAIN
- Blood clot in the lungs
- Heart attack
- Angina (heart pain)
- Breast lump

HEADACHES
- Stroke
- Migraine headache with neurological problems (blurred vision, spots, zigzag lines, weakness, difficulty speaking)
- Other headaches caused by pills
- High blood pressure

EYE PROBLEMS
- Stroke
- Blurred vision, double vision, or loss of vision
- Migraine headache with neurological problems (blurred vision, spots, zigzag lines)
- Blood clots in the eyes
- Change in shape of cornea (contacts don't fit)

SEVERE LEG PAIN
- Inflammation and blood clots of a vein in the leg

You should also return to the office if you develop severe mood swings or depression, become jaundiced (yellow-colored skin), miss 2 periods or have signs of pregnancy.

PILLS AS EMERGENCY CONTRACEPTIVES:

2 Different Approaches: Progestin-Only Pills OR Combined Pills

PROGESTIN-ONLY PILLS

Plan B

1 + 1 pill 12 hours apart OR
2 Plan B pills ASAP
after unprotected sex

20 + 20 pills 12 hours apart

Ovrette *(yellow pills)*

(Plan B and Ovrette are NOT carried
in all pharmacies. Check in advance.
Ask your pharmacy to carry Plan B

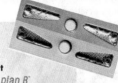

plan B®
(LEVONORGESTREL)

PLAN B

Antinausea meds not necessary ◀——

COMBINED ORAL CONTRACEPTIVES

2 + 2 pills 12 hours apart

Preven *(blue pills)* OR
Ogestrel *(white pills)* OR
Ovral *(white pills)*

(Preven Ogestrel and Ovral are NOT carried
in all pharmacies. Check in advance.)

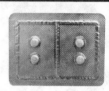

4 + 4 pills 12 hours apart
Low-Ogestrel *(white pills)*
Lo-Ovral *(white pills)*,
Levora *(white pills)* OR
Levlen *(light orange pills)* OR
Nordette *(light orange pills)* OR
Triphasil *(yellow pills)*,
Tri-Levlen *(yellow pills)* OR
Trivora *(pink pills)*

PREVEN

Have your patient take
antinausea medication an
hour before the first dose if
using any of the combined
oral contraceptives as
emergency contraception.
This is not necessary if
using Plan B.

5 + 5 pills 12 hours apart

Alesse *(pink pills)* OR
Levlite *(pink pills)* OR
Aviane *(orange pills)*